THE POSITIVE SIDE OF CANCER

My faith and hope journey with breast
cancer

DEBBIE LOESEL STANTON

Copyright © 2017 by Debbie Loesel Stanton

GRATEFUL ACKNOWLEDGMENTS

This book was professionally edited by Leanne Sype, who caught the vision for this book. Without her skilled assistance and encouragement, this book would not have gone beyond a rough draft.

Interior design by Julie Pfeifer. She is a very loving and patient teacher who offered her assistance at just the right time.

Portrait by Daniel Peyton. I am blown away by his talent, and I will never be able to thank him enough.

I received and used many helpful suggestions from my beta readers. Though I do not mention them by name, they know that they have my unflagging gratitude for the part they played in this project.

All photos courtesy of GraphicStock except for author's photo on About the Author page and Daniel Peyton's portrait of the author in the Bald is Beautiful chapter.

NAMES USED IN THIS BOOK

The names of authors Ken Barr and Tom Lucas are used with permission. Besides Debbie Loesel Stanton, all other names are fictitious to ensure privacy.

ISBN-13: 978-1975870010 (CreateSpace-Assigned)
ISBN-10: 1975870018

SECTION ONE

MY CHRONOLOGICAL JOURNEY
Traveling from Point A to Point B

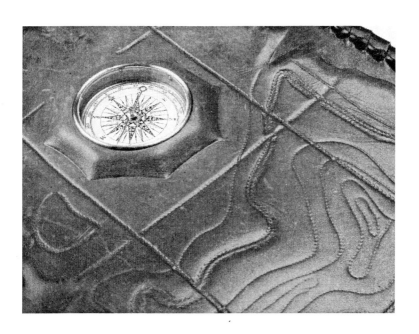

MY LETTER TO CLARA

On August 24, 1994, my only sibling, Clara, died of uterine cancer. On August 24, 2009, I was diagnosed with breast cancer. I wrote Clara a memorial letter three years later about my feelings for her and her untimely death. I also told her about my cancer and having fought for both of us. It helped me a great deal to write that letter, but I do believe August 24th each year will be a bittersweet day for me.

August 24, 2012

Dear Clara,

If you could be with me now, I would tell you that I don't believe in talking to the dead. But, in this case, I feel that if I talk to you through a letter, I will be able to celebrate the life you had and also the fact that you are still with me in spirit. When I close my eyes, I used to see you and me, Mom and Dad; there is only me now. There are three, actually black spaces where you guys used to be. But, I am glad you are in heaven now – of that I am sure – and that you are living a serenely glorious life. In fact, you are really LIVING and not just existing. I asked the Lord how you were doing one day in my prayers. I got the answer, "She's finally **HAPPY** now." What a wonderful concept!

I never was mad at God for your death at the tender age of 39. I figured God had his reasons, and his ways are much higher than my ways.

2

Although you were very sick at the end -- and in and out of a coma – I had a wonderful time with you at the hospital. I talked to you and sang to you; that's the first time my singing voice ever cracked. You yourself croaked out the words: "You sound fine." Dear Clara, you were misguided but very sweet!

When you could finally sit up in bed, I put my back up against yours so you could remain upright (I think the cancer had gotten to your bones). I slept in a cot next to your bed all night, if sleeping is what you could call it. I remember refusing to go home, and the next morning when your pastor paid you a visit, he found me there sleeping and promptly took me home to Mom's apartment.

I laugh now at the spectacle I must have been. I was still in my bathrobe and fuzzy slippers, taking the elevator and walking in the parking lot, but I didn't care. You and your life were much more important to me than looking all spiffy with every hair in place.

I have warm memories of your hospital stay. One night (early on, before your coma) you insisted to Mom and me that we get a bunch of groceries to bring back to the room. I, of course, obliged, even though we all knew that you weren't able to eat solid foods anymore. The grocery list went something like this: fig bars, punch, pizza, and MY favorite, apricot nectar. I remember thinking "This sounds like a party!" (Of course, we missed Dad being there. He was already in heaven at that point. But I just recall how jolly he was at get-togethers, with those twinkles in his eyes.) Just today I realized: You were trying to have your own swan song and say goodbye in a happy atmosphere. Bless you, Clara!

When I came back to the hospital, Mom said you went to sleep right after I left. I believe we just left the food for the staff to eat. You went into a coma the next day, but the day after that I dutifully read a letter to you that my friend Paul, and later husband, had written so he could say goodbye. I had heard that people in comas can hear what you're saying, so I made sure I read the letter and kept my words positive as well. Paul had done such a good job with writing the letter, and it was very hard for me to get through reading it out loud without losing it. Mom interrupted me and said, "Look, Debbie!" and you were reaching for my hand. I think it was during the part of the letter where Paul was telling you to reach for God's hand because you are His child and He was on your side. Or, maybe you were saying "yes" to salvation from God? Trying to comfort me, maybe? I don't know, but that was another tender moment.

One or two days later you died in the morning. Your pastor visited me and Mom at the hospital, and he wanted to pray with us. I was so exhausted, and Mom and I had already done so much praying together. We had kept praying for God to take you home to him – but you were stubborn. You held on for two days longer than someone with kidney failure would…To think of praying even more, especially since you had already passed, seemed like asking for the impossible. I told the pastor okay, we could pray. I sat down on the linoleum floor, right where I had been standing. No sense of decorum or sitting nicely, but I didn't care! I was internally angry that I had just lost my only sibling, and outwardly? I'm sure I was crabby. The day before, the nurse had told me and mom that we couldn't come in your room to see you yet. If we weren't immediate family, then who was?! That really got me steamed.

As Mom and I were leaving the hospital that day, I stopped into the family waiting room on your floor. I think those people were supposed to be there, because I had a message to give them. Just picture me standing on a soapbox – that's how I felt. No stage fright! Ha! I didn't care what they thought when I said: "If you have someone in your family that hasn't heard you tell them how you feel about them, make sure to tell them right away. Because one life, one young or old life, can be taken away in the blink of an eye!" Clara, I told you I love you when we got you to the hospital, the morning after I flew in at 11:00 p.m. Maybe I didn't say it enough. But from the day you left and after, I have told hundreds of people that bit of advice. It's like I want to get my message out there -- now – and to everyone!

I am different than you remember me. Ever since that night, I don't act the part of little sister anymore. I have confidence now and try to stand tall. I don't let myself get bullied or bossed around. Ever since the nurses didn't treat you well enough, in my humble opinion, I received the confidence that you always had.

That night I was driving west, next to the Bay, when I saw the most incredible, beautiful sunset I had ever seen. It wasn't a typical Midwestern sunset with muted colors. This one looked like it actually belonged in Hawaii, with its streaks of your favorite color, hot pink, against purples, blues, and yellows. I had the sensation that somehow God was putting

His blessing on the day and on your departure to Him. My heart ached like crazy losing you, but the sunset gave me hope that the God who created nature and such beauty was totally capable of giving you a very wonderful new home.

Three years ago on your 15th anniversary of going to Heaven, I got my own diagnosis of cancer. When I realized what day it was, August 24th, I knew then that I would be fighting my cancer battle for me AND for you. Your cancer had progressed so rapidly that you didn't have a chance to fight. Well, I would fight for both of us, I told myself.

And I have. There are only a few bad memories of my cancer journey; the rest was wonderful. I am writing a book centered on the positive part about cancer because before I had cancer, I never realized there could be something positive about that word or experience.

Well, Honey, it turns out that you received what I call "The Ultimate Healing" – the chance to go home to God. Some people get that kind of healing, and some get healed so they can live more years on earth. Either way, it's all in God's loving hands. I am glad I will see you again in Heaven.

I love you, you precious girl!

Your little sis,

Debb

P.S. I wish I could hug you one more time. Knowing that I will see you again in Heaven doesn't take away my loss…but it's a start.

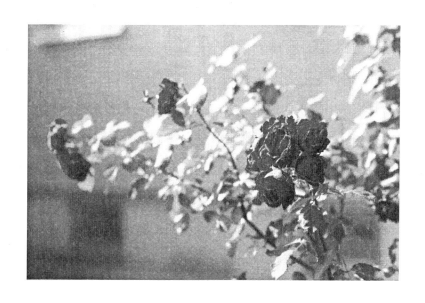

DIAGNOSIS

I had missed my yearly mammogram by three months. Next week, I told myself, *you need to make that appointment!* Before I could make the appointment, I was standing in front of my closet one Sunday morning, buttoning up my shirt. My hand brushed against my right breast. I felt a lump. Uh-oh! Fortunately for me and my stress level, my doctor's appointment center was staffed on Sundays, so I was able to make an appointment at his office for a couple days out. To follow protocol, I first had to see him so he could verify the lump's presence before I would be able to see an oncologist. *Why can't I go to the breast health center, where the oncologists are, for an appointment right now? Aren't we always told to get a lump checked out immediately? Besides, I know there's a lump, so let's just cut to the chase!*

Soon after, the oncology team performed a biopsy on my lump. They were trying to collect some fluid from under the skin in order to test it for cancer. The breast offered not one drop. Stubborn thing! After finally getting the sample they needed, I was given the instruction to wait for the oncologist to call me with the results in two days. If I had not heard anything by five o'clock, I could call them.

At three o'clock on the second day I just could not wait any longer. A very nice female oncologist answered my call. She said, "Unfortunately, yes, you do have breast cancer in your right breast."

My voice shook a little bit as we made arrangements for me to be seen again. The scared feeling I would get making speeches in high school rushed back; I was also in mild shock. I say *mild* because I was still functioning albeit in a dazed manner. Me – now having breast cancer?

I knew my cancer would be life-changing, and I knew I needed support. I was a single woman with no family nearby. Good friends, as I gratefully learned later, became my life support.

I prayed, "Okay, Lord, so what is my first step? Can you please guide me through this?" I spent time holding my two cats and talking to them. Then I started making phone calls. I could hear the shock in my friends and family's voices. I can't remember what my friends told me, other than they were sorry to hear my news. I do know that talking with these friends helped me a great deal. Whatever they said was a beautiful lifeline for my distress. I was numb with shock, but all I heard myself say was, *Okay – here we go!* Somehow, deep in my soul, I must have been ready to take this journey.

I had liked medical shows on TV since I was a kid, and I've always been curious. I suppose that is why I didn't put off seeing a doctor when I felt the lump. I didn't want to end up like my sister, who I'm quite sure could have seen her doctor earlier. What you don't know can hurt you. Give yourself a fighting chance and get checked out.

GUTSY

About a week after hearing the diagnosis, a friend of mine, Savannah, the mother of my godson, met me at the hospital where we were to talk with my oncology surgeon. The surgeon was a very nice person, but not the same lady who had given me my diagnosis over the phone.

"So, when do you want to have your lumpectomy?" Doctor said.

My relationship with God, then and now, was a secure constant in my life. I did not ask Him specifically about my treatment, but I believe that God usually speaks to me through my intuition – my gut feelings.

I wanted my breasts gone! I was endowed with large breasts – the exact size is not important to know – yet my personality did not depend on their presence. Fortunately they were in proportion to my body size, whether thin or overweight. Yet, my breasts had gained me unwanted attention. I was okay with and ready for a no-breast-life! There was also a fear of the cancer returning if I had just a lumpectomy because of the history of cancer in my mother and sister. Because of this history and a suspicious ultrasound, six years earlier I had demanded, and received, a total hysterectomy which also took my ovaries.

"Lumpectomy! I don't want the lump removed, I want my breasts taken off. Yes, both of them!" I responded rather vehemently before the doctor could ask me to clarify. I had to restrain myself from snapping my fingers and pointing at her as if scolding: I definitely surprised myself at being gutsy for the first time in my life.

Fortunately, my doctor didn't fight me on my decision, although she did think a bilateral (double) mastectomy was unnecessary.

Several times during the appointment, Doctor asked me to reconsider my decision. "You only need a lumpectomy, you know." But, I couldn't and wouldn't be swayed. I believe God knew what was ahead and spoke through me. That's the only way I can explain my courage. I held firm, even when Doctor said, "Oh, but you have such beautiful breasts!" Gag! Even though the doctor was female, my face turned pink. I felt terribly noticeable, almost ashamed, sitting on the exam table wearing just a thin paper robe!

Ha! I nearly said aloud. I had always wanted to be "flat" on top, and now I could be!

Doctor was going to allow me three or four days to think about my decision. Still, I remained secure in the knowledge that I had made the right decision.

Savannah, the friend who was with me in the appointment, is a little lady with red hair and a fiery spirit. 'Bold' would be a good middle name for her. She was always the one with the courage, but even she was surprised at my answer. She said she would have said the same thing as I did – take 'em both – but such determination and knowledge of what I want, she had never seen in me before.

It turned out my request for a double mastectomy was indeed the correct one. During surgery, the doctor also checked the "clean" breast. She found cancer had started in it, too. Sometimes only radiation is required, sometimes just chemotherapy (chemo), or even both: each case is unique. In my situation, I needed just chemo. If I had just had a lumpectomy, I would have eventually had to have a total of two chemo programs and two mastectomies. No no, no thank you. One of either of those things was enough!

During surgery the doctors could readily see the tumor and whether it had spread into my system. My breast cancer was staged, or noted, as Stage One, the most treatable stage. The size of the lump was a little under two centimeters, like a marble. The cancer was invasive and aggressive but had not gone outside the lymph nodes yet, so my case was pretty simple. I am still very glad I got it taken care of right away.

Do you know that breast cancer occurs in men, too, making up one percent of all breast cancer cases? Breast cancer in men is often found later than in women. I heartily recommend that women stay regular with their yearly mammograms. I also believe that self-examination on a monthly basis is a good idea for everyone.

Don't let anyone minimize your concerns. Stand up for what you believe.

If you notice anything different about your body, please get it checked out immediately. Waiting will not make the problem go away. Earlier detection makes for a better prognosis!

PORT, PROSTHETICS, AND PRIORITIES

Chemotherapy began for me on October 1, 2009.

MY PORT

I was to receive a port (port-a-catheter) because the inner veins in my elbows like to roll and hide and be generally uncooperative with blood draws. This "condition" would make receiving my medicine, chemo, very difficult. I thought about the word "port" much more than I thought about chemo. I had never heard of a port except as something at the edge of the sea. I was more intrigued by how a port works than I was frightened of chemo.

About three weeks after my double mastectomy, I had outpatient surgery to have the port planted in my chest under the skin. This little gadget was the entry point for my chemo drugs. The chemo nurse just administered what felt like a small shot into my port each time I came in to the cancer center.

Normally a port is placed on the right side of the chest, but because my lymph gland sample had been taken from my right side, the port had to be put on the left, closer to the heart. I'm sure the surgery was pretty intricate for that reason.

I was in pain for about three days after the port was implanted. I couldn't move my body an inch without noticing and feeling my new port site. Pretty soon the little round lump under my skin was as familiar to me as any other body part. I got used to it, even the feeling of something tight being in my chest.

I had my port removed about a month after my final chemo treatment. My doctor gave me permission to decide when the port would be removed. I was told that I could leave it in, in case I should need more chemo drugs. I would just have to come in regularly to have the port flushed with a saline solution. I chose to have it removed instead of waiting longer. I felt this girl would not need any more chemo: Again my gut instinct was correct. Remember what I said about trusting your gut?

PROSTHETICS

Between my bilateral mastectomy, my port surgeries, an appointment to be fitted for prosthetic breasts, and a genetic-based interview, I had a multitude of appointments scheduled for the hospital and cancer center. I went back to work just three weeks after the mastectomy. I was really tired!

Genetic counseling is offered to all cancer patients at my hospital. I begged to be able to see the geneticist much, much later, after I was done with chemo. Wish granted!

I wore my prosthetics for approximately one day, just two hours the first time and again for my wedding day a couple years later. They made me too warm. Since I didn't wear the forms much, I didn't have to endure the frustration over prosthetics that slipped around, but I can imagine I would have found something humorous in that situation.

I put the forms back in their pretty zippered cases, never to be worn again. Five years after my cancer diagnosis, I donated them back to the breast center at my hospital. They were just thrilled to receive them, because one of their staff made it a part of her job to deliver forms to underprivileged women in Mexico. That is exactly what I wished the outcome to be!

PRIORITIES

At the beginning of my journey I had thought that I would be able to continue the online writing class I was taking. I was halfway through the two-year course, and I didn't want to postpone finishing it. I figured I could keep going just like I had resumed working full-time. That is where I was wrong: I couldn't work, write, and keep my chemo appointments, so I got permission from my professor to hold off on finishing the course until I fully recovered. I finished the course a year after my chemo was finished.

When I had cancer, I realized that a big life change had to occur: I had to let go of my commitments and priorities, except work, so that I could concentrate on healing. This meant allowing myself to get more rest, even though at times this made me feel guilty and "lazy." It was another part of being my own advocate and standing up for what I needed and dismissing, for a time, what I didn't need to spend time doing.

> Sometimes your looks and priorities change, but that is par for the course. Remember, YOU get to decide what you want to do.

CHEMOTHERAPY

October is National Breast Cancer Awareness Month and the month I began my chemo October 1, 2009. In total I had twelve months' worth of chemo and a preventative adjunct medicine called Herceptin. My type of breast cancer, HER2 negative, called for Herceptin instead of Tamoxifen, a drug that some breast cancer survivors take orally for five years after cancer treatment has concluded.

My chemo days were painless. I usually wore a V-necked, easier-to-get-to-the-port-that-way, pink shirt, both as a way to brighten up the day, but also as a way to acknowledge that something important was getting done here: healing. Pink is the color of the United States' Cancer Awareness Month. Are you aware that the color pink means joy?

During the first month of chemo, the nurse had to wear something that looked like a space suit, goggles, and gloves. This was to prevent the medicine from accidentally splashing on her. The medicine container was even labeled "toxic." I knew that if it was toxic, it would kill the cancer.

Going to my chemo treatments was like going to my own personal spa. While there, I could really rest and relax.

The nurse always put me in a private treatment room if one was available. It contained an adjustable bed with freshly-warmed sheets. The bed could be adjusted to a comfortable position, depending on whether I wanted to sit up after being hooked up to the medicine or if I wanted to lie flat and sleep through the whole session. I usually napped through my entire session. I was glad that even hooked up to my medicine, I could sleep on my sides!

The chemo sessions lasted between one and three hours. My nurse, Melanie, would hook me up to my medicine, bring a heated flannel sheet to cover me, close the blinds on the tiny window in the door, turn off the light, and close the door. A dark, quiet haven.

There were also a TV and DVDs to watch and a CD player. Once in a while I would have the nurse put in my favorite CD to listen to as I drifted off to sleep, but usually I would opt to just rest in silence. These sessions were a way I could get my rest since I was working full-time while going through cancer. I cherished these quiet times. I didn't need someone in the room with me. It was the only time I had to really get some good rest. Though exhausted constantly, I still had problems sleeping. Getting chemo was like a switch turned on inside of me that said, "Okay, Debbie, you can rest now!"

Over the course of my 12-month treatment and adjunctive therapy, I grew attached to Melanie and the other nurses; my oncologist was also a tremendous source of love and encouragement. This is how my body heals: with positive emotional support. I usually went to my chemo sessions alone, because the hospital is located near my worksite, and I always walked back to my car feeling cherished and whole. Getting chemo was a time and place filled with acceptance, unconditional love and unlimited support and help when I needed it. The staff there were in the right job for them, because they took the time to be kind and to listen. Wouldn't it be nice if all of us were like this? I felt that there, I could be myself. I could just be me, something I had not learned was okay until that point.

On my last day of chemo treatment, the staff presented me with a certificate for having gone through my treatment program. It was beautifully decorated and signed by all my providers along with supportive comments. I still have it on my bulletin board at home! Melanie even wrote how she was looking forward to reading my future books. Unfortunately, Melanie no longer works for that hospital, but I hope someday she can find this, my first book, and smile!

The staff who loved and cared for me became my friends. Even though I would see my oncologist again and see my nurses in the hallways at the cancer clinic, I knew that our relationship would change. This celebratory day also included a few happy tears.

> I had not known what to expect from chemo, but it turned out to be a wonderfully beautiful experience, better than I could have expected. I did not know that through cancer, I would come to a place in my life where I could feel glad to be me and a person in my own right without having to try to be like other people. I would get to feel completely loved and safe. What freedom! What a gift!

WARM FUZZIES AND THE 'I LOVE BOOBIES' BRACELET

My godson Kenny and his brothers, Theo and Tyler, all wore pink rubber bracelets supporting breast cancer survivors, in honor of me. I think of all three of these young men as my nephews, for I love them very much.

Tyler got in trouble at his school because his bracelet said "I like boobies." The teacher didn't like the language on it and confiscated it the very moment she saw Tyler wearing it. Poor Tyler, he was just being a supportive nephew, and he didn't care what other people thought. He was in grade school at the time, and he was little, but his heart was so big and loving!

I felt bad his teacher couldn't have been more understanding, because there was a special reason those particular words were on the bracelet. Thanks anyway, Tyler!

I got another positive, warm fuzzy feeling from the boys' mother, my friend Savannah. In a music store at the mall, Savannah and I were wasting time until a movie started nearby. Across the store two teen boys were making fun of my bald head. Savannah marched over to the boys and said, "Listen! How would you like it if your mom had cancer? Leave my friend alone!" They mumbled "sorry" to her and ran out of the store. If I was the Velveteen Rabbit in that store, I would have become "real" at that very moment. I felt so loved.

When the incident at the mall happened, I had been taking my treatments and happily working. But when the two teenagers made fun of me, my peace disappeared, and I felt bullied. I felt hurt and depressed until Savannah spoke to the teens in the store. If she had not done what she did, I might have gone into a funk which could have lasted a long time. The oomph that Savannah provided would last until the end of my experience. Her bundle of love and peace offered me the determination to keep on fighting. Thanks, Savannah, for being my advocate!

Similar to Savannah is any person or people who advocate for their cancer-survivor friends or family. The support and love they show strengthens the friendship, educates onlookers on how to treat people lovingly, and gives tremendous fighting power to the survivor. The strength in my inner person is still inside me today. I thank God and my advocates for this treasure.

> I think advocacy for others is so important. To this day, I want to be like Savannah and her family.

HAIR REGROWTH IN FOUR-FOUR TIME

Having my hair grow back was a process that I or even Dr. Jay couldn't control. Hair regrowth mattered to me because I was beginning to be a content person and appreciate the things I used to take for granted. My regrowth can best be summarized in four stages.

SOFT, NON-WHITE BRISTLES

When my hair started coming back, it was very dark blonde; it was a shade darker than my natural hair color had turned out to be. Unlike my previous hair, no highlights or lowlights were present. Since I had just turned 51 when cancer hit, I was thinking a head full of white hair would be fun. I did not want silver hair. I definitely wanted white! It goes to show that you can't place an order for your new hair color like you can order your favorite salad dressing flavor!

I loved the feeling of my new hair. Though very short, the bristles felt like duck's down or baby hair. It reminded me of greeting cards with velveteen covers. Yes – I indulged the people who wanted to touch my "duck down" and feel how soft it was.

What interested me most about my new hair was my hairline. Having had Barbie dolls when I was little, I likened my hairline to Barbie's boyfriend, Ken's. My hair grew into a crew cut, with a hairline that was completely straight across.

THE JFK HAIRDO

When my Ken-doll hairdo gave way to longer hair growth, I was amazed. At the time, I thought I resembled President John F. Kennedy. My hair was thick like when I was younger, just like his, and very wavy. I was glad to welcome back thick and wavy hair, and it remained the same dark-blonde color that my bristles had been.

FUNKY HORIZONTAL

Then the change happened. My hair stopped growing longer, and began to grow horizontally, much like an Afro. I had fun never knowing what I would wake up to the next morning. I was just glad to have hair!

DEBBIE HAIR

My hair eventually grew vertically again, and I lost most of the curls, as well as my wish to have all-white hair: it just wasn't happening. I waited long past the recommended six-months waiting time to have my hair colored again. However, I don't get it colored very often. I don't want my scalp to be touched by bleach – my skin is already very sensitive. Nowadays, my natural hair has many shades on one head. What little amount of gray I have, I am letting it exist. It's due to the fact that I feel good to have hair at all. Once a baldie, always a thankful person, is my new motto!

My cancer journey increased my playful personality and helped me laugh about things that used to concern me such as my appearance. My hair is what I laughed at or smiled at most. To this day, sometimes (usually) my hair doesn't cooperate with my styling efforts, but that's how a lot of life works: unpredictably. So I make the best of what is, and I am glad to have hair days. Period.

Have fun with your new hair. It's going to be okay!

DEBBIE AND PAUL

Since Paul's presence kept me calm, I had nothing to fear when he was with me. We had a good friendship going.

Around the middle of my cancer journey, Paul and I became closer and went to many cancer benefits together. I just wanted to HELP people; Paul with his never-changing generous nature wanted to help cancer survivors too. Going to benefits was a part of my healing, and my relationship with Paul deepened at the same time.

In addition to going to benefits together, we were enjoying time together at my house – another unexpected gift: having Paul by my side helped me to see even more qualities in him that pleased me immensely and added to my gratefulness.

In 2010, Paul and I went to a benefit for a family whose house and dog were lost to a huge fire while they were out of town. When I saw the news story, my heart went out to them because my family had also had a house fire when I was in sixth grade. I had written to the grieving mom that she would recognize me at the benefit because I would be the bald lady.

It was on the way home from this benefit that Paul and I realized how close we had become. We admitted falling for each other in a big way. We were dating now! I wondered where this was leading, but yet I wasn't in a hurry. More and more in my life, I was able to take on a "wait and see" attitude about practically everything.

In early winter 2012 Paul proposed to me. He and I married in late autumn of the same year. My husband and I are both immensely grateful that I survived. Our relationship remains loving and solid. Out of cancer came something wonderful!

> My husband became my cloud's silver lining.

SECTION TWO

TOPICS
Items of Interest

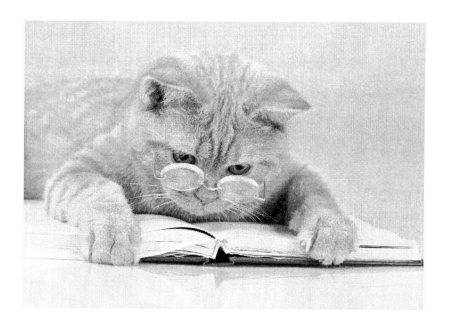

ATTITUDE

When I was walking through life with a bald head, I had amazing conversations with different people. They all went like this:

PERSON: "Debbie, how can you walk around with a smile all the time? I don't have cancer, but I'm usually frowning."

DEBBIE: "It's how I look at life, I guess. Basically I'm just glad to be alive."

In those conversations, I didn't have time to stop and think of a good answer. But, I have found that your mood or expressions really do depend on your inner life. I can choose to be grumpy or choose to be thankful. I can remember that there are more positives in my life than negatives.

You only go around once in this life. Let's see and reinforce the good and stop wasting time fretting about everything else.

> Outcomes are what they are, but positivity produces better reactions.

BADGES

I've heard of a badge of courage. There are badges for just about every good virtue or characteristic. Cancer gave me many badges. It is fascinating to me how something so ugly and so life-threatening is a harbinger of good things.

If I were to be given badges for my cancer experience, they might be the following:

Boldness

Never before have I stood up for myself so readily or not wonder what other people would think if I did. Cancer gave me the confidence to not care what other people thought of me.

Serenity

What a peace that has entered my soul and my life. As I survived cancer, it seemed possible to do anything I used to think was impossible.

Courage

I wanted to survive cancer more than anything I had wanted in my entire life. It was this mindset that helped me push through the healing process. Pain and the "what ifs" were just distractions along the way, but they didn't stop me.

Acceptance

To curl up into a ball and want to die would not have led to acceptance. Rather, I realized that in every life, trials and difficulties come which help us to grow and conquer. It was not my duty to ask "why?" but rather acknowledge that there were worse things to battle – to be a victim of violence or war, to see your child die before your eyes, or to be tortured – to name a few.

Hope

There is always hope, no matter how small, in each situation. In the many difficult times of my life, I still had hope for the future. I knew I was in the loving and caring hands of God. I began to appreciate all the research the medical community has done to find a cure; this too offered me hope. My doctor is a brilliant man with a humble and loving personality. All three things let me rest easy, and hope was born.

> Each of us, no matter what we are going through, have the ability to choose what badges we wear – how we deal with the storms in our lives. Sometimes the toughest things bring out the tools that we didn't know we had. My wish for all of us is that we don't give up but continue to pursue the good.

BALD IS BEAUTIFUL

Good communication is necessary in a conversation so all parties can understand. Sounds simple, doesn't it? Yet many people like to express themselves and only hear, rather than listen to, the other person in the conversation. Some, who I appreciate very much, really listen to who they are conversing with.

When I was bald after chemo, I was at a conference with absolutely nothing on my head, not even bristles from new hair growth. I left the conference hall to use the ladies' restroom, where I was accosted by an older woman. I say *accosted* because she was really in my face about something that didn't concern her, and she was not listening to my words.

"Oh, so you're not wearing a wig?" she started out her questioning.

Um, isn't this evident? I wanted to say.

"That's right, I choose not to," I replied sweetly.

"But don't you know that the State *has to* provide you with a wig? It's your right, you know," this only half-listening person went on.

"I don't want a wig. I don't need a wig," was my gentle rebuttal. Maybe in *her* eyes, I did need a wig.

"I don't know why you don't wear a wig. You have to let the State buy you one!"

Uh, did you not hear what I just said?

"That's alright," I stated and breezed out of the bathroom while her mouth hung open.

I think of all the information she could have gathered if she had chosen to just **listen**. It would have not taken very long; I had a simple story: She could have learned that I had tried several scarves but they were too slippery or uncomfortable. I occasionally wore hats but more often than not, it was easier just to not worry about what to put on my head. The wig was too darn scratchy, and *it was not me*.

The non-listening person would have learned that I felt I had nothing to hide. The cancer wasn't my idea, and I had nothing to be ashamed of. In fact, I had everything to be thankful for, because the baldness showed that the chemo was working. I was comfortable in my own, smooth and bald, skin!

The playful part of me wonders what it would have been like if the lady concerned about my no-wig status had fussed about my no-fake-breasts status. She might have said, "Oh, but the State HAS TO get you prosthetics!"

After that I was at another conference and got the opposite reaction.

"Oh, thank you for not wearing a wig," an older lady said to me. "I have cancer now, and I'll be able to go without a wig because you were so courageous not to."

I'm glad I could help! God bless that woman who encouraged me that day. To encourage someone with cancer is one of the nicest things you can do for them!

Did you know, there have been several French models that strut down the runways without hair? I give them my vote!

When I was growing back my hair, I got the inspiration to start a website called "The Hatless Society." It was meant to provide encouragement to chemo patients who didn't feel like wearing a hat or wig or scarf. But, I didn't know what new information I could keep putting on the website, so that idea went the way of the circular file.

Some cancer patients need to wear a hat if it is summertime and they don't want to get a sunburn on their scalp, or if it's cold out, or even if it's to keep their head warm while they sleep. It is up to them.

People who choose to be bald have many reasons, too. My main reason had been that I just wanted to be me, naturally me, whatever that looked like during this time of sickness in my life.

The important thing is to not resent bald cancer patients for "not following the rules", and not to pity them or to believe that they just want attention. Going bald, or choosing to be bald, is another of those things that just need to be accepted in a person, to "live and let live." Isn't that what we want others to do for us?

I believe that sometimes, "rules" are not rules at all, just opinions that aren't necessary for everyone to have. Opinions forced upon other people are, in fact, devious ways to trick people into being exactly what you think they "should" be like. So if it's not traffic rules and laws to keep us safe, let's not impose our rules and opinions upon others.

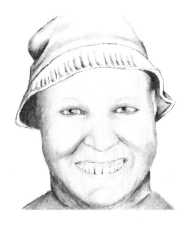

Let loving hearts become listening ears.

People don't like "should's", so let's let them form their own opinions.

BLESSINGS

I found that recalling all my blessings helped me in a big way. I didn't feel like my life was spinning out of control, because these blessings grounded me. My journey seemed pretty easy, only having two bad reactions due to the chemo medications and a blood transfusion.

There was Margaret, who took care of me at my home after surgery. There were people who sent me get-well cards, and they probably don't know how much their words meant to me. I still have the cards in a wicker basket on my hearth, because even now they provide me with so much hope – for all of life.

My friend Paul took me to my first chemo appointment, and my friend Tricia took me to chemo each time the regimen changed. When Dr. Jay and nurses were trying new medicine and didn't know if I would be able to drive myself home afterwards, Tricia was there for me. She and I even got to have lunch out on the way home, and that was a treat. Time out in public reminded me that I was still in the land of the living, and I could still have fun. Time spent with Tricia then paved the way for a wonderful friendship later on. She was no longer just a neighbor.

I received divine comforts in the form of warm flannel sheets, a nice spa-like room for chemo, comedy shows, cozy shawls and blankets, and other sweet gifts from Paul, my friends and family.

My movie pal, Molly, continued to see new movies with me monthly. This kept my spirits strong and helped us stay close. She also braved snowy, icy highways during rush hour to pick me up from my overnight stay at the hospital after the transfusion. It turned out to be 24 hours that I was hospitalized.

My schedule was grueling. I continued to work at my job full-time. Thanks to anti-nausea pills I was given during the first course of chemo, I was not sick at all. I was fortunate to be able to use my chemo sessions as restorative nap time.

Working during treatment was very good for both my financial status and emotional stability. It helped me to have something familiar from my life before cancer. It was good for me to see people every day and feel their love and support, especially since I lived alone.

Modern medicine's blessings are the research physicians and scientists have done, the financial support of many organizations and individuals to provide for that research, and powerful drugs to combat cancer. As of this writing, we have not found a cure for cancer, but I believe it's on its way.

Every cancer patient is different regarding depression and isolation. Though I was single and just living with two cats, I didn't have time to feel lonely. My friends at work and church, and my friends in my personal life, all contributed to the life-giving warmth I received in my heart, mind, body, and soul.

All the blessings I received helped keep me in a positive frame of mind. Even when feeling the need to be alone, the effects of the blessings took root in my soul as I took time to contemplate and pray. The blessings in recovery grew my peace, strength, and love, thus allowing me to feel confident in facing anything that came my way.

> Don't forget to remember your blessings, for they play a special part in your journey

I used to love to cook and bake, but writing is now my go-to activity. I wrote a "recipe" of sorts — hope you will enjoy!

RECIPE FOR RECOVERY:

Get your area ready by sitting quietly and turning the results over to the One who loves you.

Add the memories of blessings received to your stockpile of hope.

If at first your stockpile is hard to find, search and believe, and you will find it.

Sift in some new life from above along with prayers and thanks.

Strength will form. This will help you to stand firm.

Now, throw in some smiles, even if not heartfelt. (They will produce something of value even if you don't feel it's possible.)

To this mixture add the seeds of beauty seen and the oil of joy.

Work in with your hands, and don't worry if sometimes the batter seems sticky.

Now, sprinkle this recipe along your path. It will then light the way for your fellow travelers.

For best results, repeat daily. Serve up as often as needed for a life well lived. Rejoice as you give, for you will not be found lacking.

BLOOD CELL COUNTS

My doctor tested my blood levels at the beginning of each chemo session so he could be informed of my blood cell levels, which can fluctuate during chemo. The chemo medicine for each appointment can be adjusted if necessary. Sometimes despite good nutrition and other protocols in place to counter low blood cell counts, red blood cells dip too low.

During my first round of chemo, I received a Neulasta injection at the hospital every Saturday to prevent levels from getting too low. However, dipping too low happened to me – SEE Transfusion Woes.

I received half of the blood allotted to me before it was discovered that my body was rejecting the new blood. I had to stay overnight at the hospital so they could watch me closely. Fortunately, my blood levels did improve from the transfusion, and I never needed another one again.

WHAT I HAVE LEARNED SINCE THEN

Please note: I am not a health care professional. I am simply presenting what I've learned as helpful information to my readers. I do not guarantee any outcomes due to the reading of this information.

Neulasta patches, to be worn at home, are now becoming available.

Low blood cell counts are related to risk of serious complications.

FACTORS FOR KEEPING BLOOD LEVELS HIGH

Eat a balanced diet. If you do not have an appetite, please consult your doctor or oncology dietitian for help.

Do not eat raw meat or eggs.

Use an electric shaver rather than razors to prevent cuts.

Avoid germs and those who are ill.

Do not clean litter boxes, fish tanks, or bird cages.

Rest as much as you can.

WHAT DO THE BLOOD CELL COLORS MEAN?

White: These blood cells help the body to prevent infection. A low white blood count cannot fight off infections.

Red: Red blood cells carry oxygen to the body. Symptoms of low red blood cells: tiredness and being short of breath.

Blood transfusions are given for red blood cell deficiencies. Generally, they are not given for the white blood cells unless absolutely necessary.

CARE SQUADS

The first year of dealing with cancer is most critical because cancer can be stopped in its tracks, or at least grows slower the sooner it is found. Aggressive action is needed as soon as possible to give a patient a good fighting chance. For me, part of the aggressive action was identifying my team of helpers. I call them care squads: At first I wasn't aware that I would need them, but I consider myself blessed to have had them in my life during this special time.

I took my cancer journey with no parents, siblings, children, or husband – but two cats. The people in my "care squads" were my support, and in this way they became my family. I have since revised my definition of *family*. Family is the group of people who are there for you in time of need and who you would assist in their time of need. Family is made up of friends and loved ones who care for you and love you unconditionally in the same way that they love their blood families.

A large part of my healing came from how I was treated and my mindset. My mindset remained positive due to the love and comfort I received from my family, friends, and medical team. Without my friends and their little displays of love, concern, and comfort, I am sure I would have felt as if I had been sent to appointments at the cancer care center to just give up and die. These wonderful people confirmed the hope I had received in my spiritual life. They are the reason that the tears I shed during cancer recovery were those of gratefulness, only happy tears.

My Lord and Savior brought the connections together because he knew that I needed a family during cancer. Knowing I had an adopted family plus my friends helped me stay focused on recovery, and I did not have to worry – about anything.

I had a whole team of people in my corner: family, friends, and church; my oncologist and chemo nurses; volunteer staff and those providing services and shawl makers.

FAMILY, FRIENDS, AND CHURCH FAMILY

When chemo started, Paul accompanied me and sat with me in the treatment room. Wasn't that nice of him? What a comfort, what a Godsend he was and still is. It was helpful for me to know that someone was there for me, cheering me on and silently giving me lots of hope and peace.

My friend Margaret stayed with me for a little while after surgery. I was thankful for her driving me to post-op checks, the grocery store, and even the local ice cream shop. Margaret's cooking was delicious! She was also very helpful in helping me with the drains to get rid of the post-surgery fluid building up.

My neighbor down the street, Tricia, brought me to some chemo sessions, read to me when asked, and she took care of my cats for about three weeks until I was healed. Other neighbors brought me hot meals.

My coworkers held fundraisers for me, which helped a lot when my vacation and sick days, a benefit of my employment, had run out. The donations of vacation time from coworkers was really appreciated. It allowed me to have money coming in even if I had to stay home ill occasionally.

My coworkers often slipped gas cards, grocery store cards, and gifts on my desk when I wasn't looking. These helped, too! It bothered me that I couldn't thank the anonymous givers of gifts, but I sent an email to the whole department, thanking them profusely for their kindness.

I needed a lot of support during this time, because cancer and recovery was a brand new road for me to travel. I learned that it was/is okay to ask for help. My single-woman independence had to be altered momentarily. I think that was an important lesson for me to learn as well.

In a way, I was still mildly in shock at being a cancer survivor. My team gave me the necessary means to remain healthy in body, mind, and spirit.

Spiritually, every breath I took was a prayer of thanks to my God. I listened to words of comfort from people at church and meditated on verses in the Bible. I was very blessed indeed to be one person with so much love showered on her.

MY ONCOLOGIST AND CHEMO NURSES

Dr. Jay and Melanie were my favorite parts of my cancer adventure. If Dr. Jay, Melanie, other nurses, and even the receptionists had been emotionally cold toward me, I would not have survived.

Dr. Jay's temperament is perfect for his job, and he is well respected in the community. He shared his kindness and concern with me, many other patients, and supervised the oncology residents. He made it to work one Christmas Eve morning when our first blizzard-like storm of the season was happening. Dr. Jay called me personally to say don't bother coming in for my appointment; he didn't want me in an unsafe and nerve-wracking situation, and chemo could wait for a day.

About halfway through my treatment schedule I, who usually didn't complain, was falling apart. My side effects were getting to me. The side effects on top of my full-time work schedule, as well as chemo schedule, were just too much.

"I can't handle this," said I in his office, "what should I do?"

"But Debbie, you have to look at yourself," he said.

My hair was gone, and I looked like Uncle Fester from the Addams Family TV show! What did he want me to see?

"You ARE handling this. You are one of the few patients I have who work full-time and still have chemo."

I listened to his encouraging words and a few days later realized, "Yes, these symptoms too shall pass."

Dr. Jay knew how to treat me without acting like I was a number in a medical system. His wisdom and encouragement did me a world of good.

Melanie was my main chemo nurse. Oh, the fun we would have. We enjoyed talking about our families, and I begged her for stories about her two little girls. I told her I wanted to write for children. Melanie was an encouraging part of my chemo life!

She knew what I liked for my chemo sessions, and she made sure I got what I preferred each time: a dark, private room; the shades within the little door window fully shut; and the door itself closed. It was like being at a spa, and Melanie made sure I was comfortable.

Melanie was one of the reasons I felt sad when my chemo ended in the next year because a lively friendship had blossomed from a chemo experience, and I knew I wouldn't be seeing her again.

THE VOLUNTEER STAFF, PRAY-ERS AND SHAWL MAKERS

At my chemo center, volunteers came to visit the patients to see if we wanted something to drink or some hot soup or goodies. A lady masseuse would sometimes come to massage our hands and feet if we wanted.

I was also given two handmade "prayer shawls" from church, which have been used a lot, even post cancer. Soft and comforting, they were just like the hand-knitted and crocheted caps at the cancer center that were there for the patients' taking.

All the prayer chains and faithful friends who prayed for me were such a blessing. Prayers and faith were imperative for my recovery. There is definitely power in prayer, and I felt that power flood my being. I had nothing to fear except to wonder if I would have enough energy to remain working.

Some people are crafty with their hands. Savannah and her family made me a soft, pink tie-blanket with positive words in darker letters. Her mother-in-law made me my very own quilt with blues, yellows and pinks.

I've heard the saying, "God doesn't close a door without opening a window," and I believe this to be true. All these people in my cancer picture became my fathers, mothers, brothers, and sisters when I needed them the most. I am indebted to all of the people in my squads. God bless all of you who give of your heart, your time, your love, and your service to help someone in a health predicament.

Many people make up your village of health and recovery.

COMPARISONS

During my cancer recovery, people often informed me about their family members and friends who had cancer, the fact that their treatment program was longer or shorter than mine, or they made decisions opposite of the decisions I made for myself.

It's interesting that I seemed to hear these comparisons at the times that I could barely function. It was very bad timing! I remember smiling at these people who were delighted to tell me other cancer stories, but inwardly I was spacing out and planning my getaway.

God bless them all, but really, these facts were not important for me to know. Why? My case was different than anybody else's. I could not possibly have the same exact treatment plan or situation. Therefore, there is no one right way to "do" cancer. Comparing one's self to other people is not a good idea in general, but when you're talking about cancer, it's vitally important to remember this. Hopefully friends and relatives of other cancer patients will remember this as well.

> If you are the patient, don't listen when people compare you to others. If you are friends or family of a patient, don't be the one comparing. Focus on the patient! Thank you.

EMOTIONS

You may be surprised at the emotions you now feel more strongly: anger, frustration, fear, sadness. Do not worry or feel bad about them, because they are a normal part of the process.

I feel everything emotionally much more acutely than I did before cancer. Joys are very intense; I am more appreciative and thankful. When I am treated really well or I see someone else being treated well, I do get teary, even now. It's all good, though. Perhaps knowing what I could have lost makes me this way.

Each of us is born with emotions inside. We are made this way because we are human. Accept that you have emotions and remember, it's okay that they're not always pretty.

ENCOURAGEMENT

Laughter, love and joy produced from my cancer journey increased my capacity to encourage and love others. I was blessed to be given a second chance.

Is there a person in your life that could use some encouragement? Practice the skill of being encouraging to others! It's never too late to start.

Do the people you love, know that you love them? They may say they don't need to hear the words, but vocalizing how you feel about them hits the target, reinforcing feelings of love and goodwill. Building one another up is very much needed. On a basic level, it is the right thing to do.

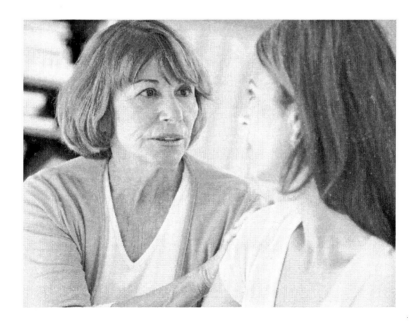

FAITH

I've believed in God since childhood and have always believed He loves me. Sometimes I thought He was the only one who loved me: it was this knowledge that began my faith.

I sensed His presence during a family house fire in elementary school that nearly took our whole house. I did NOT sense His presence when I nearly drowned as a youngster – but sometimes anxiety hid Him from me in different situations. Faith, however, remained.

My sister passed away from uterine cancer when she was 39 and I was 36. I was a midlife orphan by my mid-40s. By this time, I was ready to be done with the growing list of sad times in my life, yet I acknowledged that maybe God was preparing me for something. *It must be a doozy*, I reasoned.

I'd say breast cancer was a doozy! As when my sister died, I did not blame God. I did not have to assign blame for my situation – if indeed I actually could. With cancer, I felt I sat in the hollow of God's hand, safe within His care. I remained positive and inspired, not because I am a super-human person who can deal with anything; I had been given a whole storehouse of blessings. Where had they all come from, if not from God? This is what I am like even all these years later.

God gave me a profound gratitude for life, more real and heartfelt than ever before. When I prayed for comfort and relief, He answered my prayers through all the blessings I wrote about in the Blessings chapter.

Because of faith, I could see these blessings as not bandages, but the giving of life, over and over each day. Lamentations 3:22-23 says, "Because of the Lord's great love we are not consumed, for his compassions never fail. They are new every morning; great is your faithfulness." (New International Version Bible – NIV)

My faith has grown not because I wanted good cancer recovery, but because of what I experienced through cancer recovery, all of which I was and still am thankful for. My God never left me, nor has he ever forsaken me. I believe he orchestrated everything, chemo included, for all aspects of my care to enable me to see life after cancer. Thank you, God, for being a miracle worker!

FLU SHOTS

It's a general rule that if you have an ongoing condition like diabetes, or if you are elderly or work with the elderly, sick people, or children, you should have a yearly flu shot.

I am not a doctor, but if you asked for my opinion, I would add flu shots to the "cancer survivor's needs" list. However, those persons allergic to eggs are usually advised not to have flu shots because of the ingredients in the shots.

A cancer patient can get pretty run down when their blood levels are low. A flu shot prevents getting even more run down which can really hamper the patient. During my cancer year I was glad I had a shot because when I needed a blood transfusion and could hardly keep my work schedule, I was glad that something additional like the flu would not bring me down further.

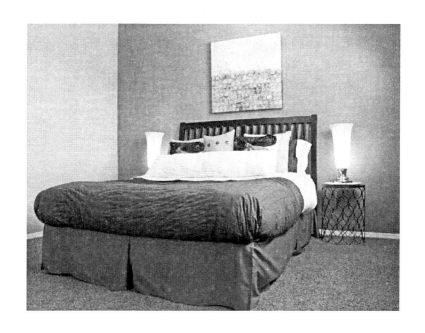

FOOD

Lean animal protein or plant-based protein helps the body to produce new, clean cells. It's a good building block for your system.

A good supply of fruits and vegetables provide vitamins that your body needs. I did not change my diet at all, and I regret not doing so. I'm sure I would have had more energy during my recovery if my diet had been better.

Do you need to go organic? If going organic does not strain your food budget too much, then yes, I'd recommend it. If you can't, just concentrate on getting good balanced nutrition.

If your appetite is low or absent right now, please call your cancer center, oncology nurse or dietitian. They can provide help.

Sometimes a cancer patient notices that food tastes funny or has a metallic taste. This too can be brought up to your professional.

A good tip for anybody is: try to eat less processed food. Sticking to food the way nature provides it is better for your system. I have a fun way of remembering this: If you don't see a doughnut tree or cookie bush in nature, you can be sure your body doesn't need it!

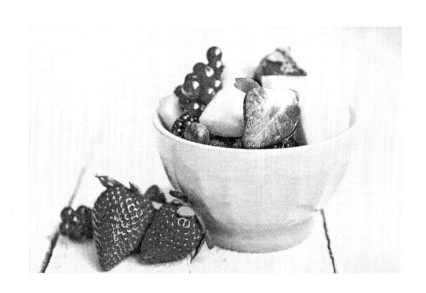

MY FREEDOM COLOR: PINK

I consider the color pink to be my freedom color.

When I was a little girl, my mother dressed me in pink all the time because it was HER favorite color. When I was a teenager, I decided to "hate" the color pink simply because my mother loved it, and I was mad at her for no reason in particular other than I was a teenager. As a teen, I also had my first cocktail: a "Pink Lady." I found it disgusting!

Outside of the color pink, I was brought up in the old-school way of thinking about colors and fashion. No white after Labor Day unless it's cream or winter white. Purses should be in dark colors if it's winter time.

I also used to have insecurities about what people thought of my choices regarding colors in clothing and interior decorating, my clothing style, and pretty much everything about me. I had not yet taken God's promise of love into my heart. I wonder after all these years why it was so important for me to care what others thought of me. It was the only way I had been taught.

The old-school rules took a flying leap out of my life once I had cancer. Since I was given the gift of life and recovery, I wanted to express myself fully. No more bowing down to "you should do this," personal rules, or caring what other people thought. Today, I realize that I am my own person, and I am supposed to be different from others, because that's what makes me the person I was created to be.

When I was diagnosed in 2009, the color pink appeared in my closet more often. Too bad my mom had passed away by this time and couldn't see me wear pink again! As my inner transformation gained speed, I embraced my new-found boldness and bought a bright, magenta-pink wool coat for the Midwest winters, with mittens and hat to match. This was only the beginning!

One day, I spied a must-have-it, hot pink purse at the local Target department store. It was the jackpot of handbags, ladies! A beautiful, just-the-right-size-and-number-of-pockets-and-zippers, hot pink, buttery-soft leather purse!

I decided that even though most people don't use bright-colored-purses during winter, I could and would. Besides, it wasn't even in the sale section, so the store wasn't begging people to buy their off-season purses. Apparently hot pink was now "appropriate" in winter. Even if it wasn't okay for other folks, I would claim it okay for me! As I purchased the purse, I wished that Clara was still alive, since I know she would have adored this purse, too.

There was a day when I wore hot pink jeans and a pink tee-shirt to work. I smiled when coworkers said maybe they would have to wear their sunglasses indoors to avoid the brightness. With my smile that others have described as bright, I felt like one hot mama…

> Finding freedom is the ability to not bow down to what the Jones's are doing, buying or thinking.

Funny enough, my favorite color is still not pink; it's pastel yellow, with aqua, turquoise and red coming in as close seconds. I love all kinds of colors more fondly than before my battle with cancer. I no longer shy away from bright colors, especially pink. To me, they say "Life"! Cancer has given me a voice, so to speak. It is a statement of freedom to be me.

FUN THERAPY

I recommend taking a little time and engaging in something you really enjoy if energy permits. Reading a book you can get lost in. Going back to an old hobby that you loved, like painting. Coloring in the coloring books that are out there for adults. Taking a nap that would feel really good. Listening to music without having to do anything else but *be*.

Fill your cup with things you like to do – and fill it full!

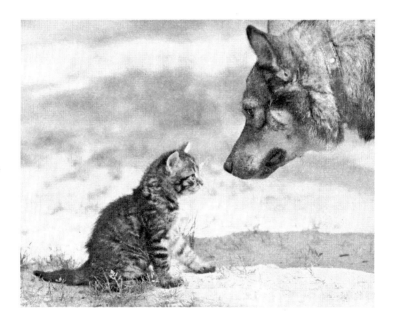

GUILT

Sometimes I feel guilty that while I survived, other people have died from cancer. Other cancer survivors have told me they feel the same way.

This guilt is not necessary, but it still pops up every now and again. I have to remember that every case is different. Every cancer occurrence, whether simple or very complicated, takes some strength and courage to get through. I can remind myself that I am not in control of others' outcomes, and for my case, I did what I had to do.

I have also heard people say that cancer is a punishment from God. Please do not believe this really false guilt. If someone dares to guilt you, I would want you to just walk away. You don't need that negativity!

I am alive for a reason, and I can celebrate this by making each day of my life a day well lived.

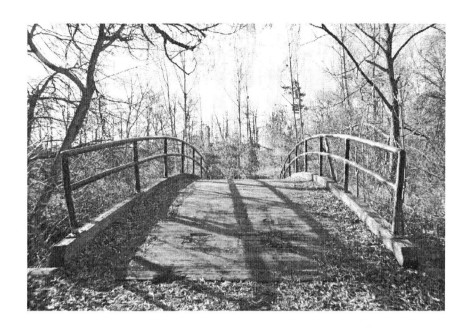

HOLIDAYS DURING CANCER RECOVERY

I learned this in a grief group I had attended: when the holidays arrive, give yourself permission to change up your normal ways of celebrating, or consider not celebrating until next year. You may not feel like participating in the things you did before. That is perfectly acceptable; simple can be sensible and just as meaningful.

I remember that a friend of mine brought my Christmas tree and ornaments up from the storage closet in my garage and decorated my tree for me. Then I didn't feel like I was missing anything. I remember going to church alone on Christmas Day. That turned out to be okay, as the red chili pepper kerchief I wore on my head made other people smile.

Let this be the only expectation you have for yourself – and hopefully others' expectations for you: do what you absolutely have to and disregard the rest. If you normally bake a holiday treat that everyone asks for, remember that this is an out-of-the-ordinary year, and next year is soon enough for that treat. You have now entered into a period of rest and recuperation that you need.

About Christmas trees…they have always been my favorite part of Christmas, even more than the holiday food and presents. My friend mentioned above was so nice to put her needs aside and put my tree up for me. My world didn't fall apart when someone else put up my tree. I was pleasantly surprised to find that last year, when my husband and I didn't feel like decorating for Christmas, not even putting up a tree, we found out it was okay to leave the house as is. It felt a little empty, but otherwise we had a great Christmas. I am here to say that it is okay not to follow your same traditions year after year!

If you need help and ask for it as I have suggested, you may get a "no" from someone. No problem. The next person you ask will probably be able to say "yes". Most people who offer their help really do want to be contacted so they can find out what you need most. Let them help you.

> This may be the year to try a new holiday tradition or don't follow a tradition at all.

INSENSITIVITY

When a person is not listening to a cancer survivor, or anyone, really, in a conversation, you can be sure there's some insensitivity present. Remember the lady who told me I had to wear a wig?

It's a fact that people will say something inappropriate or off the wall out of embarrassment or if they have no idea what to say. I think if you focus on listening to the patient, you can think of something kind to say that would relate. We cancer survivors are just hoping for acceptance, and sometimes that means hearing opinions that don't resemble yours.

When I was first in recovery, I saw many, many looks of fright at my bald head, as if their seeing me would somehow give them their own cancer, or at the least remind them of their own mortality. I also saw many gazes averted when they saw me coming. Perhaps my not wearing a wig seemed shameful. However, the shame was on them.

There were a few times when someone would ask me how I was, and I mistakenly started to answer because I thought they really wanted to know. Not! After two words into my answer, they'd interrupt me and tell me how their family member was doing.

Someone told me that I should style my hair, when literally that would be impossible. How can someone style a butch cut, which is what my duck's down bristles looked like? Hair that is too short to comb is too short to hold a style, right?

The classic response that you've probably all heard is "I know JUST what you mean," when they have never been in your situation. Maybe they are kind people who don't mean any harm, but they somehow get sidetracked and say something like that. All you can do is pray for patience.

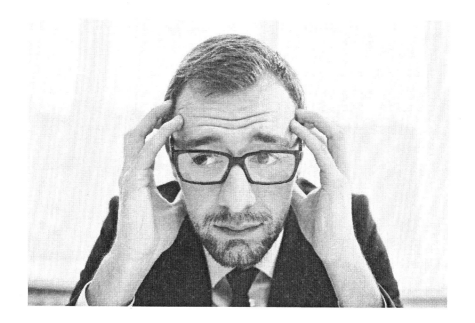

LAUGH

Occasionally I felt down or overwhelmed. That is when I had to consciously choose to look for joy and find the humorous details in life. Usually a health crisis or bad event brings about anything BUT joy and humor.

Laughter and humor do not hide in closets and pop out when needed. I had to seek them out. Learning to purposely laugh was a way to improve my cancer recovery. Laughing has the ability to take me away from my present circumstances, much like a good book. Laughter is a good reminder that life still goes on.

I found ways to either see the humor in my situation or sought out things that I knew would make me laugh or smile:

Laughing at *Laurel and Hardy* or any comedy show that felt good both internally and externally.

Funny videos on TV, especially the ones with kittens, puppies, and babies.

Old black-and-white movies from the 1940s that showed clothing and hairdos not seen in our present day; I could also practice speaking English with an accent by repeating what the actors said.

Sometimes life seems absurd or downright laughable. It helps to know that this is not a black and white world. There is always a colorful personality or situation that can evoke a smile or a laugh, which is healing for the soul!

Rather than getting mad at terrible drivers, I started to pray for these people that I didn't know. Once I believed I wasn't going to die, I started to realize that traffic patterns weren't the most important thing in my life. I didn't have to get mad anymore about trivial matters. I could laugh at the people who turn right from a left turn lane!

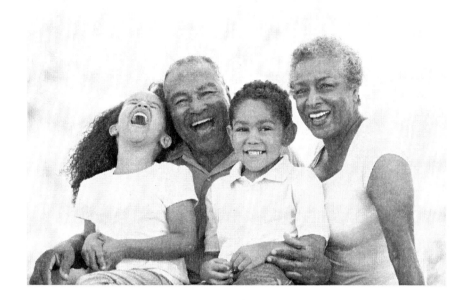

LIFE AFTER CANCER

There were days both in my recovery and afterwards that I felt so glad to be alive. I looked at little things in life with a new perspective.

TRAFFIC

The bad driving habits of people on the freeway were not important. They were amusing or irritating but not important. The fact that I was able to drive and still have a job to go to – now that was important! Questions like "Why are some people so odd or cruel? Why do they act stupidly?" no longer mattered. There were more important things to do: live life in a thankful and simple manner and in my heart believe people are more valuable than things.

I'm noticing other people's bad driving habits these days, but I still remember the new perspective I have learned in cancer recovery: it's easier to let go of mundane irritations when I sense their unimportance.

MORNING AND EVENING

My love for morning has returned since surviving cancer. Sometimes I won't even sleep in on weekends. It is especially fun to drive into the sunrise or to see it from my kitchen table. My God, who I call the Master Artist, paints a different sunrise each morning. No two sunrises are alike, just as each of us is created differently. Each sunrise heralds another feeling of peace that washes hope into my being. Hope that I have a brilliant future ahead of me, and I need only live each day, with thanks, to find it. Hope that since I recovered from cancer, I can do just about anything I set my mind to. In fact, the book you are reading is the "anything" I set my mind to. There is hope that even bad things can turn out in a good way if I'm open to the possibilities. I feel the hope that there will always be so many things to be thankful for.

I've always enjoyed sunsets and the way they look like paintings in the sky. I do love evening walks under a star-studded, moon-enhanced sky, though I am no night owl. I'm beginning to really admire the evening, even though at the end of the day, my energy is completely spent. My concentration and energy still run low; however, if my day has been lived well, twilight brings my body and heart peace and calm.

Darkness in the outdoors announces the end of another day, yet offers its own kind of hope. Hope that I'm getting close to the morning and renewal of mind, body, and spirit. The sure knowledge that I will again be blessed, and kept watch over and protected by the One who made my life possible not once but twice.

> The glass-half-full person sees what is there, and the glass-half-empty person notices what is missing.

MEDICINES

Herceptin – I was given this in the form of chemo after my last regular chemo was over with. This was given to me because my condition, HER2 negative, cannot take *Tamoxifen* which some patients take. Herceptin is an adjunctive type of therapy used as preventative maintenance.

Neulasta – this is a shot given once a week to help keep good blood levels.

PALLIATIVE CARE

It is true that cancer patients who undergo chemo have to receive enough medicine to practically kill their bodies, because this is what kills the cancer. If people choose to have palliative care, and use "natural" methods to heal instead of Western medicine, so be it.

Be careful with alternative treatments, though. A long time ago I had an acquaintance who moved back to her home hundreds of miles away. We found out about six months later that she did this so she could eat or drink nothing but carrot juice after receiving a breast cancer diagnosis. She believed with her whole heart that she would be healed with that one regimen. She didn't want anyone to tell her not to go the carrots route.

My friend basically had gone home to die: within three weeks she was gone. It angers me that this friend's ignorance, maybe a fear of using Western medicine, and probably shame, claimed a good person's life. I did my research and decided to go with what my doctor recommended, and I am very thankful I did. I believe that God works through doctors and nurses. I am alive today because I received chemo.

REST

Rest can recharge your body's processes and give you more energy. No longer is rest a luxury; it is very necessary. Rest can be different than sleeping. Resting is quieting your mind, heart and body. It is doing quiet activities that are relaxing. One thing I didn't try was putting together a good jigsaw puzzle with a backdrop of quiet music. Try to remember that rest is a state of "being" more than "doing." Naps are excellent ways to relax. During my treatment, I was in a total state of rest during my appointments. It was so nice to take naps and not have insomnia at night. Now I don't dare take a nap if I am working the next day.

Rest is always recommended, whether you're in treatment or not. When we're healthy, it's so tempting to skip having adequate rest, saying we don't have time or it's not that important. However, when your body is trying to heal, it needs rest. As much as you can muster!

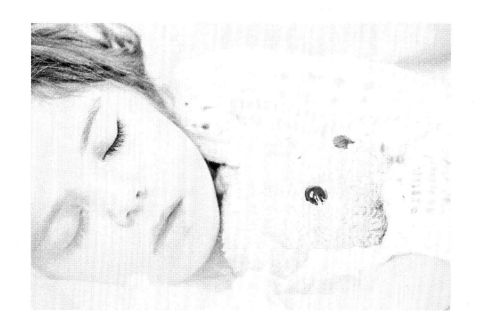

MY SIDE EFFECTS DURING CHEMO

Some people have the same side effects as I did, and some do not. They may have side effects that I never had to deal with. Every single person is different. Accept the reactions of your own body with grace. Be kind to yourself! Remember there is nothing to be ashamed about, whether it is regarding your choice to not wear a wig, using prosthetics or not, working or not working during cancer treatment, or even the fact you have/had cancer.

Some of the side effects I had anticipated from chemo never surfaced. For example, I didn't experience nausea or vomiting. Within my chemo "cocktails" was medicine to prevent nausea. I drank lots and lots of water after each session which I think helped me to avoid sickness. However, during one four-week period of time, I lost both my appetite and 20 pounds. However, I did not have to worry about the weight loss. I already had more than enough weight to sustain me!

CHEMO – FIRST COURSE

My body had strange reactions to the poison, as most patients do. Most of these reactions were during the first course of therapy, when the most toxic medicines were administered. Some of the symptoms were hoarseness in my voice and I couldn't sing right anymore, red and peeling palms, jumping nerves in my legs and feet, and a constant runny nose. The nails on my big toes fell off. Surprisingly, that didn't hurt.

CHEMO BRAIN

A side effect that began midway during chemo and persists in me to some degree even now is what other people have named "chemo brain" or "brain fog." It was at its worst in the beginning, with fuzzy thinking and forgetfulness. Most people get over this eventually.

ENERGY

How much energy a cancer patient does or doesn't have is subjective. Hopefully patients get their strength back quickly, but there is no one "average" time in which you can expect energy to return. In my case, I never fully got my energy back. I used to put myself down for that and relentlessly push myself to do the quantity of activities and chores I had done before. I don't do so anymore. It is not a punishment to have low energy after a major illness. It does not mean I am lazy. I am just glad to still be here and writing.

EXHAUSTION

I experienced severe tiredness from working full-time through all the treatments and discomfort of side effects. Even now, I wonder how I was able to keep up with such a schedule. One possible explanation is the fact that when you're fighting for your life, you just do what you have to do, and you don't question.

HAIR LOSS

Even though I knew there would be side effects, with each new symptom I said, "What? You've got to be kidding!"

Everything felt like a surprise, except hair loss which led to baldness. THAT I was prepared for.

I was told I would lose my hair, but that didn't happen until awhile after the loss was predicted. A good thing coming out of a bad side effect: I didn't mind losing my hair. Having hair or not did not define me as a person. I knew it was part and parcel of having my sort of chemo. People with certain other types of cancer or chemo don't lose their hair.

SEE the Hair Regrowth in Four-Four Time chapter that describes the stages I went through.

To make the transition from hair to baldness easier, I first got a very short haircut. Three weeks later I had my head shaved, to be as close to bald as I could come. That was a momentous occasion, thanks to my dear friend Jeannie. I was feeling terrible at work that day, and a friend outside of work called me and made demands of my time later that day. I was forced to agree to do something I did not want to do. Jeannie knew this, and as soon as we were both done working for the day, she drove me to see her beautician after work, who buzzed all my hair off. That appointment sure helped me to feel better.

My neighbor at the time loaned me her old red wig. I started itching immediately and so hardly wore it. When I did, it was for an elderly lady I hadn't seen in a long time – I didn't want to scare her! After returning the wig to my neighbor, who said I should still wear it, I wore scarves of cotton only, because the silky scarves slid around too much, and caps, which were of cotton but still annoyed me, did not stay on my head very long. It didn't take me long to go without anything on my head, except when outside in the winter. What freedom! Being bald in public is not for everyone; it was just my choice. As I understood it, Margaret told me if I didn't wear a wig, it would be like I was asking for sympathy. She did not know me well enough to know that I would never do that, much like I can't pretend I'm someone else. I wouldn't make a good actress! I just stood my ground and went without anything on my head. Of course, many people verbalized their opposition to my practice. SEE the Bald is Beautiful chapter.

There are some people in this world who are insensitive or act scared of a person with cancer. The phrase "live and let live" definitely has meaning for me now!

LUNG INFECTION

One of my courses of therapy predicted that a very few people might expect lung problems. Being the sensitive-to-medication person that I am, I did get a lung infection. I was taken off that course of chemo and put on Prednisone for several weeks to help with breathing and my coughing.

A GOOD side effect to Prednisone: I had the strength of an ox. I was moving furniture in most rooms of my house, freely, easily, and without assistance. My major accomplishment was moving my heavy oak computer desk across my home office to the other side of the room. There is no way I could do that now, especially by myself!

What got me through was God's miraculous strength he gave me and my attitude of wanting to fight this cancer. All I had to do was accept the side effects and trust that these would be temporary. They were markers on the road to recovery.

I trusted God with the spiritual part of my journey. He is such a great Teacher! I trusted my heart when thinking about the quality of life I had before cancer and what I wanted it to be after.

No two cancer stories are alike, not even within families. There is no guide that will accurately predict everything that will come up in your journey.

In my recovery, all my side effects combined to form something that would change my life in such a positive way. Positives about cancer? Who'd have known?

MY SIDE EFFECTS NOW

I battle insomnia here and there. I try to keep a good sleep schedule as often as I can, and I try to get some exercise every day. I tend to sleep better if I've gotten up and moved during the day – but not too close to bedtime.

The lack of energy I still have is probably related to the insomnia. I am working on taking care of myself in the best ways possible to see if my energy will come back.

The chemo course that made my legs and feet restless left me a remnant of that. Many years after chemo was finished, my feet would burn, tingle, and shoot pains – similar to diabetic neuropathy, from what I hear. Then it happened so often that I got maybe two hours, total, of sleep per night. I called in sick to work the mornings after those occurrences, because it would be unsafe for me to drive a car after just two hours of sleep. After I was told that I was missing too much work, I called a podiatry office that specializes in dealing with neuropathy. I told the doctor on the phone that something just has to be done, that I couldn't miss any more work! Then, twice a week for eight weeks, I would travel from my job downtown to the doctor's clinic three highways away to get treatments. I don't like driving downtown, but this time I didn't have a choice.

I also took vitamin supplements custom-tailored to my situation.

One year after finishing therapy, my neuropathy symptoms returned, although much less severely. I am now in my second run of therapy, and I still take my supplements.

Since finishing the first course, more data has been obtained, and I believe this will make my new course of therapy more effective.

TALK THERAPY

Cancer survival can sometimes put you in a slump. You want to feel better emotionally, but it's difficult to stay on top of everything, much less concentrate on taking care of yourself.

My cancer center had a psychotherapist available to help with cancer issues and feelings. I never visited that person, but I do encourage people to see a therapist if they want to have an objective listener. A therapist can help you come up with ways to counteract sadness, fear, anger, and frustrations. These are all normal parts of surviving cancer, especially at first.

There is a cancer survivors' group at my hospital. I never attended because I was too tired from work and all my appointments, but I hear that it is a wonderful place to go and talk with other people who are going through the same thing as you. Support at any and all levels is an excellent resource!

Sometimes it's hard to talk with family and friends because they tend to want to solve all your problems quickly. Known to "mother" my friends sometimes, I know that I would want to help cancer patients in this way too.

Family and friends sometimes give advice that may or may not reflect the actual situation. It is not their job to manage your emotions, and I would like you to stay away from feeling responsible to take care of someone else that's hurting at the moment. I give you permission to do whatever would help you.

I don't like to talk on the phone. If you're like me, you could ask people to text or email you, and then you can check back with them when you're ready. Which reminds me…it's totally okay to finish a meal without answering the phone! That's what voice mail is for.

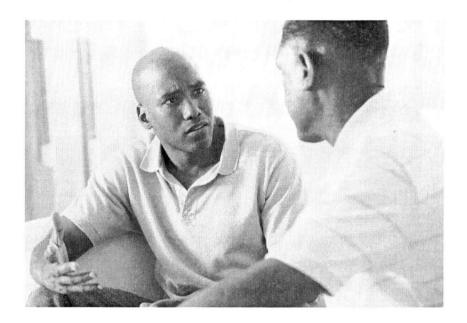

TEARS THAT WERE HAPPY

I was always a person who found it easier to cry for other people – in sad movies, and for mistreated people and animals – than it was to cry for myself.

Even when I got the news of my cancer diagnosis over the telephone, my eyes welled up with tears and my voice was a bit shaky, but I didn't weep.

Now, however, I easily cry when I am treated in a very kind manner, because I am so thankful, or when I see people being kind and helpful to others. Going through cancer gave me an appreciation for love, family, loyal friends, joy, times of solitude, peace, kindness, faith, and hope. Thankfulness flows out of my being through streams of tears – happy tears.

Many cancer survivors say they are thankful for their cancer. I feel the same way because without cancer, my emotions might have remained stifled and unexplored. Cancer was a harsh teacher, but a good one in helping me to discover who I am and how to express how I feel. For me, I found happy tears in suffering. I have learned it is okay to shed tears. It is the happy tears I cherish most.

As much as I never imagined I would have happy tears, the same held true for cancer. I never thought I would get cancer, even though my mother and sister had each had uterine cancer, and my sister died from it. When something "funny" was going on with my reproductive system, I proactively had a complete hysterectomy. *There*, I thought, *now I don't have that risk. Cancer, you have to stay away!*

But cancer still found its way to my breasts. I was surprised to learn that breast cancer can be, but isn't always, a familial thing. No one in my immediate family (parents/siblings) had ever had breast cancer.

The good Lord, in all His wisdom, allowed cancer to arrive at my door at just the right time. It wasn't good timing in my opinion, that's for sure, but there is a time and season for everything. I had lost my sister to cancer when she was only 39 years old, and my parents had already passed on. By now, I was a single woman with a mortgage. Did I really need this cancer now? Really?

I didn't fall apart, just asked God, "Okay, so what is my first step? Will you help me through this?" His answer to me was felt in my heart as a big, resounding YES.

My cancer brought me joy and more faith. Sure, cancer was tough to go through, but I learned how to appreciate all of life. I might not have been that fortunate if I had not had the cancer. To live a happy life was another of my dreams, and now it is being lived every day. Life is meant to be lived with love, grace, patience, and hope. As in most of life but not always, we come out of dangerous situations. The Lord certainly is present, even when/if you don't talk to Him much!

Thank you, God.

TRANSFUSION WOES

There was only one time when I did not have a positive outlook during my journey. It was the most influential time in my life that changed me.

I was in the hospital, scheduled to get a blood transfusion because my levels were dipping dangerously low. My friend Rhonda had driven me in case I felt woozy afterwards and wouldn't be able to drive home.

Rather than being put in my regular, private infusion room, I was asked to sit in a recliner in the general transfusion area.

"Ooh, I'll have an audience," I quipped.

Rhonda and I had quite an interesting conversation going, and then she got stir-crazy. She decided to take a walk through the hospital. Knowing I often slept through my treatments, I told her it was perfectly acceptable for her to take a break, and she should have an enjoyable time on her walk.

One bag of blood had been imparted to my ailing body, and the second bag had been started. That's when my turmoil began.

I began to get so warm, I was threatening to take off my [only] top, and now I wasn't joking. I had developed a fever because within about 10 minutes I was freezing cold. I actually DEMANDED that the nurses give me *several* flannel sheets fresh from the heater.

When Rhonda returned much later, she found me wound as tight as a mummy with all my flannel sheets and covered completely with only my eyes, nose and mouth peeking out.

The nurse asked me, "Do you want to tell her, or should I?" I was so out of it that Rhonda started to cry.

The nurse said, "Debbie has had a severe allergic reaction to the new blood she received. We need to keep her overnight, I'm sorry."

This was one treatment I didn't sleep through. This, right here and now, was the moment that changed my life forever. I felt like I was dying. With my temperature rising and falling during the transfusion, I was very sick. I was so scared, but I knew that if I survived I was going to look at life differently and act accordingly. My life did not flash before my eyes, but even without that happening, I knew deep within me that life is a very beautiful thing, and its precious value was not something to throw away. Life is not a commodity whose value fluctuates depending on positive or negative events surrounding us.

I had been an encouraging person by nature, but that night in my hospital room, I launched my new intent to appreciate life and encourage others even more. I made the nurse laugh, and I encouraged her to share all about her family. I told her she made a difference and she should love herself because she is special. She was on the verge of tears.

Later that evening my pastor and his wife came to visit me. I regaled them with several tales, and as they left, it seemed that they walked away with a spring in their steps that wasn't there when they arrived. Laughter was definitely present, and I believe it healed me from my allergic reaction.

WATER

Lots of water keeps dehydration away, which is another problem you don't want to add to your cancer condition.

Water is vital for so many processes in the body, such as keeping body temperature normal.

If you can't stand the taste of tap water, there are alternatives. Try carbonated water or spring water. I personally don't like fizzy water, but that's just me.

Trying some lemon or lime in your water can give it a bit of taste.

Milk and juice count as a fluid serving, too, although coffee does not because it is dehydrating.

If you can get used to tea, the many flavors of decaffeinated or herbal tea are a good water substitute. Vitamin water comes in flavors and different qualities, such as Vitamin B for energy.

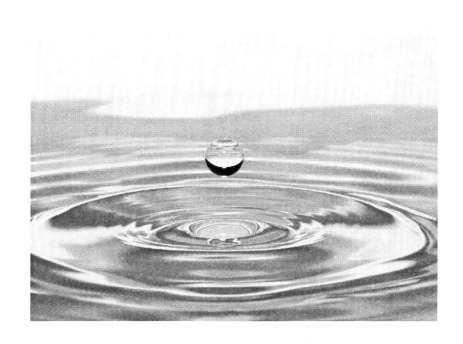

WRITING

I think I was born a writer. As a seven-year-old, I wrote what I was thankful for in the inside cover of a Bobbsey Twins book. Later, I treated my books as though they were gold, never writing in them and always using a bookmark! Then as an older child, I wrote little stories. I made a good start on my first book at age 12 – a fiction book for pre-teens. As a teen and ever since, I've written poems.

"You should write in a journal every day" was advice I heard from people, educators, and columnists. Journal writing was hit and miss for me. I didn't feel like it sometimes, so the journal would often sit lonely on my shelf waiting for the next round of inspiration.

When I got cancer, writing was the last thing I wanted to do. Reading, a part of being a writer, was nearly impossible too. I felt like I had lost my identity.

On the other side of cancer, a nice surprise awaited me. I graduated from my writing course and started journaling more, not as a "have to" but "want to."

Almost three years to the day of my cancer survivorship, I read a poetry book written by Ken Barr. I found it on Amazon when I was in a bad place, and it was like a breath of fresh air. I was impressed that Ken received reader comments on his books and that he answered these comments, so I reviewed some of his books later on. Later I found his blog. This was my first discovery into the world of blogging, and the sense of community within the blogging arena really appealed to me. I started my first blog, at the time named "The Sunshine Factor," and eventually started additional blogs. One of them was set up and made to be excellent by the lovely person who professionally edited the book you are reading!

I visited a blog written by Tom Lucas, this blog being so fascinating that I soon reached out to him. I was thrilled that he was the very first person to follow me on my first two blogs, and he has turned out to be a writing mentor to me. The fact that he put his first book out on Amazon was so amazing to me. I was so happy to have a small part in his book launch! I credit both Tom and Ken for encouraging me, in their own ways, to put this book on Amazon.

Then I had the good fortune of being asked to be one of four co-hostesses of a blog hop, where once a week, many people would submit a story according to the prompts given by the co-hostesses. That got me into writing a story every week; later when the blog hop ended, I put a feature into my blog to imitate the process that brought me so much joy. I "met" two great gals from the U.K. through this, and they wrote many stories for my blog.

I don't write weekly stories anymore, but I plan to get back to it. I've been told that when you find the main passion in your life, you need to spend 10 minutes a day doing that. So…in the days ahead, I will be writing at least 10 minutes a day.

My passion of writing was confirmed for me when I sat down to write one Saturday. Many hours later, I had not stopped for lunch or dinner, that's how excited and happy I was! For me to skip a meal, without being sick, is huge!

I started a list of the books besides this cancer book and stories that I'd like to write. The list was lost in my computer crash, but I remember most of them. It is my dream that someday, all of them will be written.

The ideas keep coming. I think that had I not had the experience of cancer to draw from, my creativity would not have popped out and into my writing when it did. Up until the point of my cancer journey starting, my life was fairly non-descript, with few mountains and valleys. Cancer turned that all around because now there were a lot of things I wanted to communicate to the world. Gratitude. Joy. Love. Peace. Changing as a person. Surprises and shocks, both bad and good. Acceptance. Contentment. I wanted to make something of my life, now that it had been returned to me.

My writing career helps me to express myself and gives me a platform for my inner self to have a voice and be playful.

I have a very vivid imagination, so I sometimes speak and write in a way that makes people laugh. I no longer believe in being prim and proper at all times. No longer do I try to be perfect. It's a well-known, yet less-accepted fact, that no one is perfect. No one has to be. No one can be. To strive for perfection is to make yourself nuts.

Cancer turned out to be a gift because once I got through it, no longer did the opinions and demands of others matter so much. I embraced the idea that I can LIVE my own life. I live it for Jesus my Healer and myself.

Writing has given me the confidence to love and appreciate myself and know that it's okay to be ME. I am continuously blown away by how life gets sweeter and sweeter, by the day. When I write and journal, the blessings are somehow amplified; I can see and appreciate them more.

SECTION THREE

ADVICE
For the Patient

Here are some things from my experience and education that are important for the patient to know. I've also included a section for family and friends as a way to help their loved one in the best ways possible.

As with everything, carefully weigh each tip to see if it pertains to your situation. It is not wise to believe everything you hear or read!

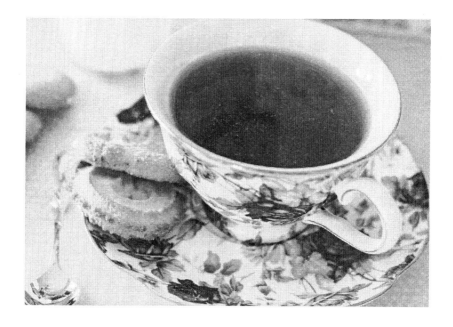

ADVICE FROM STRANGERS

I'm sure you've heard of or experienced being a pregnant woman in an elevator and a stranger comes up to her and starts patting her belly. Not appropriate, but strangers never ask permission first. That is because they act first, then think.

This is very similar to an experience I had, and mine had to do with not wearing makeup. The bank teller who dealt with me did not know me, yet she kept hounding me for not wearing makeup. She said that with no breasts now, I needed to look feminine.

"Oh, I think I still look like a girl. I don't want to wear makeup," I replied.

"But don't you want to look nice?" she further irritated me.

"Yes, but I'm not concerned. Going natural is fine." And with that, I left the bank and soon after closed my account there.

The audacity of that bank teller! Did she nominate herself makeup police or expert? Apparently, she was thrusting her views of what SHE would do onto a stranger who did not need her opinion. Don't sparkling eyes and a ready smile count for anything? And I wore feminine clothes! I felt a little guilty of being lazy after I talked to that woman, but thankfully that didn't last long! The problem was entirely on the other woman.

Perhaps I have some readers who would say that I was too sensitive, that the woman was only trying to help me. I don't consider unsolicited advice as helpful. From experience, I know that when I don't please people with my choices and preferences, and am told that I do everything wrong and am not given credit for being able to think for myself, it's pretty frustrating. It feels like they can't see that I have any amount of value. Maybe they can't see any value, but I know it's there. God made me the way he made me for a reason. Therefore, I can be confident and content.

There is one thing I could have done differently. I wouldn't have needed to give her the reasoning behind my decision not to wear makeup. I did not owe this person an explanation. Some people, like the lady who insisted that I wear a wig, would not listen to my explanation anyway.

> I've become used to just walking away if people harass me or if a conversation becomes toxic. Who needs it?

SAYING NO

Treat yourself well and defend yourself if necessary. You deserve to be treated as well as you would treat your best friend.

I've heard it said that you train others how to treat you. Cancer is NOT the time to practice people-pleasing habits, but rather to advocate for your own needs. If ever there is a time to say NO when you have to, this is it!

From experience, I know it is hard to say no sometimes. But you can do it! Say it without guilt – which may take a little practice. Even if it takes physical effort to say one word, say it: no.

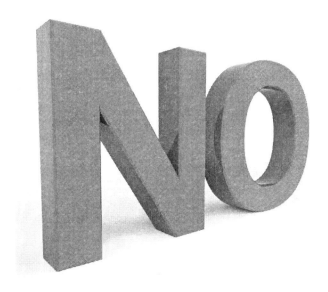

STUFF YOU HAVE TO DO

Remember that as a cancer patient, you have a right to call the shots. If you are too tired to do what you normally do, and this is practically a given, learn to feel okay asking for help. You don't have to feel obligated to act as if you're in your pre-cancer life.

Earlier in my life, before cancer, I felt like I needed to ask permission to take an hour each day for myself and do what I wanted. Once someone gave me permission, I felt much better. The guilt was gone!

In case you are like me, I hereby give you permission to do what you need to and to delegate or delete the rest.

It is also alright to say no to requests: do only the minimum and take it from there.

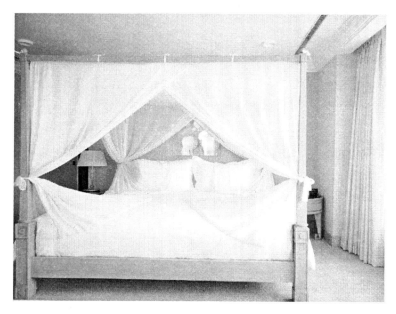

PREPARING FOR SURGERY

Make or have made for you meals for your freezer to be used after surgery. You will probably receive some meals from family and friends, but if the recovery period is long, it's good to have a backup.

Let others help you and give you moral support. You don't have to play the Lone Ranger unless you want to.

Make your home surroundings as comfortable as possible. Have your home cleaned so that being there will be a pleasure. Secure throw rugs so they won't slide around and trip someone.

Get caught up on your laundry.

Think of what you may need and make it easily available. Plenty of reading material, music, and blankets for the sofa are helpful. Buying plenty of tissues, toilet paper, and pet food and other necessities now is a good idea.

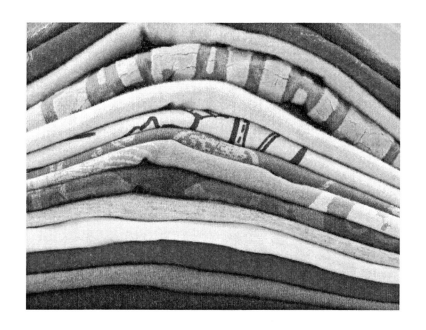

AFTER SURGERY

In your hospital room after surgery: if there is a large crowd of people to spend time with you, don't let them stay too long: they will understand.

You need to say "enough is enough" when you need to rest.

When you are at home after surgery, you need to hold back from your previous duties and abilities. I give you permission to retire from things for a while: housework, child care, pet care, sports, school and committee work. Consider yourself to be in a new kind of womb, where you will be gaining new clean cells that replace the old, diseased and poisoned from chemo or radiation ones.

Let someone help you for once; don't let your pride get in the way. People want to help! Remember that right now, you and your health are top priority.

You deserve to get well and take good care of yourself; if not for you, then for your loved ones.

Just let yourself float along while you're resting and realize that this is an entirely different situation than living an everyday life. You are a miracle that needs strength to make yourself so.

You are a cancer survivor who needs your strength even when you feel fine and don't think you need more. Believe me, you do.

Remember: you are the one in control, and if you have a caregiver who is not patient and loving and doesn't let you think for yourself, then THEY can retire from their caregiver post and let someone else take care of you.

There will be times when you think you don't need a caregiver, and if medically stable, you're probably right. I am just asking you to postpone training for the next marathon until you have felt really well for a long period of time.

I urge you to soak up all the loving care you can, since there is nothing negative about that.

Strive for positive, sunny thoughts; skip the evening news if it stresses you out, or read a condensed version online.

Put on some good relaxation music or if you love to sing, some decent lyrics. Try some comedy movies or *Laurel and Hardy* or whatever makes you feel good. Anything that will help you laugh and smile is the ammunition I advise.

Most of all – rest up as much as you can in the way that YOU find relaxing.

Here is what I personally noticed:

I needed patience with myself and others. I realized that people don't understand because they are not in my shoes. I took well-intentioned advice with a grain of salt, but I received it with grace.

You can trust your care team who will be guiding you through the whole thing.

Don't be afraid to ask for and show gratitude for help.

Don't waste time because life is precious and goes by so fast.

While life is going so fast, remember to be mindful of what is going on, in you and around you.

This, too, shall pass.

God is for me and with me, contrary to what the situation looks like.

Remember I am rooting for you. I may not know you, but I still care.

For Family and Friends

COMMUNICATING WITH THE CANCER PATIENT

Please dole out your advice only to the people who ask you for it.

Don't use the classic response of words that say, "I know JUST what you mean," especially if you haven't been in their situation.

There is no need to feel embarrassed if you don't know what to say. A good thing to do is simply smile.

Please do not ask someone how they are if you don't really want to know.

Do not tell the cancer survivor that they had it better or worse than your friend or relative. Each person's story is unique and should not be used for comparisons.

LISTENING

Whatever the topic of conversation, I have learned that listening is a special gift that can be so healing. We need to practice listening in every situation, because it is a sign of respect.

You are talking to someone for a reason. Do not plan what you can say next, while their voice is heard in the background. Bring the person to the front of your mind, and dismiss what you wanted to say. There will be time for everyone to say what they need to, so we don't have to be selfish about who gets to speak first. It's no fun to talk to someone who is totally distracted and not listening to you.

Do not assume you know what the other person will say or how they will react. Get to know them better by really listening to their words. I am sure it will be a real gift to them!

SECTION FOUR

DEVOTIONALS

Thoughts and prayers about what survivors go through sometimes

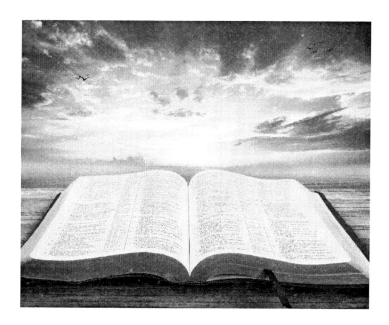

WALKING BY FAITH, NOT SIGHT

"But those who trust in the Lord will find new strength. They will soar high on wings like eagles. They will run and not grow weary. They will walk and not faint." Isaiah 40:31 New Living Translation (NLT)

Recovery from surgery and then chemo and/or radiation, or treatment and then surgery, produces exhaustion in short order. Besides getting over the surgery, there is the treatment that for a time takes the last bit of normalcy from our bodies.

Some of us also go through emotional distress – some or all of the following – anxiety, depression, and fear. That takes our energy from us, too. Much of the fight is fought in our minds, as well. We can pray, and just as likely, and maybe at the same time, we worry about the time we have to take off from work, or about our children, where will the money come from, or if we will indeed survive.

That is a lot of things to think on. But there is somebody, God, who wants to walk right beside us. If we decide to trust him that he's got this situation under control, we gain some strength – all because of who he is. He does not always bring healing right away, or even in a way that we can recognize, but it's there just the same. That is where faith comes in. We can't see God but believe that he is there.

"For we live by faith, not by sight." 2 Corinthians 5:7 New International Version (NIV)

But what if we're not sure we believe in him? Or what if we are mad at God for "giving us" cancer? Is he still God, and can he handle it if we're unsure?

God knows we are human and that sometimes we are slow to trust or believe. He understands this about us and loves us regardless.

God does not give us cancer or any illness, nor does he punish us. Because of the fallen state of this world that he created, things just happen. He doesn't give us illness, but he allows it. He uses many things in our lives that are terrible or problems that don't show up with an evident reason. He weaves them all, the good with the bad, into the tapestry of our lives, and we later may see the wisdom of why things happened as or when they did.

What does he think of me when I am mad at him? He doesn't love you any less. Because he is God, and his character is perfect love, God is absolutely unable to disconnect his love for us.

There is nothing we can do to earn his help or his love. Those things are automatic for him and are there for the asking – he loves us that much.

God's authority and power make him God. The state of our faith, or lack of it, does not make God any less God. He can handle anything. The Creator of the universe yearns to be close to us, as simple as that. He is motivated by love, even for those who don't love him back.

The future, especially as a cancer survivor, may look bleak. We may not receive healing here on earth…our days left may not be many, but when the soul in our body goes to heaven, to me THAT is what I call "The Great Healing."

If we are healed here, life still won't be perfect. We'll still have our failings, our successes, joys and sorrows. But the kind of life we can live, if we trust that he is at our side, will be better than we could ever expect.

"For I know the plans I have for you," declares the Lord, "plans to prosper you and not to harm you, plans to give you hope and a future." Jeremiah 29:11 New International Version (NIV)

PRAYER:

God, help me to believe that you love me despite my faults and shortcomings, even if I don't entirely believe that you exist. Please give me faith so I can believe. And thank you for loving me. Amen.

DISREGARDING PEOPLE'S JUDGMENTS OF ME

"Aren't five sparrows sold for two pennies? Yet not one of them is forgotten in God's sight. Indeed, the hairs of your head are all counted. Don't be afraid, you are worth more than many sparrows!" Luke 12:6-7 HCSB Study Bible

After cancer, I learned not to care about what others thought of me. I love the verse above because God, whom I consider to be all-knowing, is the one whose opinion of me I believe.

While in recovery, though, it was very hurtful to hear criticism, especially if the person was in my face about it. I also had a hard time with feeling unheard by those who perhaps meant well but wanted to have their own agenda carried out. Sometimes it was really hard for other people to hear me say "no" or "I prefer to do it (or think) differently."

"I have loved you with an everlasting love…" Jeremiah 31:3b HCSB Study Bible

God does not hurt me; I believe that he would not be able to.

I've even had another cancer survivor make fun of the scar I have from the port that was in my body for a time. It was an invalid judgment, but hurtful nonetheless. To me, that scar represents the help I received from chemo. I don't cover it up because frankly, there's nothing wrong with having a scar that gave me my life back. To that person, it represented a scar that was ugly and one that didn't heal in the same way as theirs.

Judgments are made against people all the time. I am trying to practice forgiveness now and yes, it is difficult. If you are going through this same kind of thing, you are not alone. Know for sure that I understand you.

"Do not fear, for I have redeemed you; I have summoned you by name; you are mine." Isaiah 43:1b New International Version (NIV)

Since God calls me by my name, I can trust and believe that he does love me and that I am redeemed and whole. That knowledge, if I choose to remind myself of it, will keep me feeling much better about myself because I know who I belong to. That's a whole lot better than the internal conflict I have when I am given unreasonable demands and expectations from others.

PRAYER:

God, please forgive these people who hurt me, because they probably didn't know what they were doing. Forgive me for being critical of others and judging them – I too am guilty. Help me to be quick to forgive those who hurt me and slow to remember injustices done. Help us all to have and wear compassion on our sleeves, as compassion is what is lacking all around us. Amen.

I CAN'T STAND HOW I LOOK

"Since you are precious and honored in my sight, and because I love you…" Isaiah 43:4a New International Version (NIV)

Though eventually I chose not to wear a wig, I didn't always approve of my looks during cancer recovery. Even now, every so often I am critical of my looks, and I have to remember the above verse. Being loved by God Almighty is a far more beautiful quality than what somebody looks like. Value is on the inside!

"The Lord does not look at the things people look at. People look at the outward appearance, but the Lord looks at the heart." 1 Samuel 16:7b New International Version (NIV)

I think due to the beauty and youth-driven society we live in, it is easy to be concerned with our appearance. I say "Don't dress like a slouch when you go to work," but otherwise, I don't worry about my appearance or notice new wrinkles. I could care less about what the new fashions are. There are far more important things in this life, like the fact that I have been given another day to live. And my creator approves of me, wholeheartedly.

PRAYER:

Lord, please help me to accept myself and to see myself through your eyes. Thank you for accepting me just as I am.

Help me to have grace in my heart for myself and others. Please add to my heart love and compassion. Amen.

VERSES FROM SAMUEL

I found some excellent verses in the Bible that I took the liberty to paraphrase; parenthetical text is from my own thoughts. This passage describes my cancer journey perfectly:

From 2 Samuel 22:17-20 New International Version (NIV):

"He reached down from on high and took hold of me; he drew me out of deep waters (Illness, fear).

He rescued me from my powerful enemy (cancer), from my foes (fear, side effects, depression), who were too strong for me.

They (cancer, anger, fear, depression, side effects) confronted me in the day of my disaster,

But the Lord was my support (He also appeared in human form through other people whom I call angels).

He brought me out into a spacious place (cancer-free life);

He rescued me because he delighted in me (through his grace I have been plucked from the hands of death)."

There are some persons who receive death and then the gift of Heaven as the Ultimate Healing. Whether we live or die, God loves us each so dearly. I do not deserve the grace he gave and gives me.

SECTION FIVE

PRAYERS AND POEMS

Writings about cancer

There are many times during cancer and treatment that a cancer patient or their family and friends would like to pray. Other than "A Cancer Patient's Prayer," which I wrote for myself, I have written these prayers not as my own, but to represent different types of cancer situations. The situations mentioned here are fictitious and not written about anyone I know. I offer them in hopes that they will be helpful to you.

Since praying can take many forms, I've also included poetry that can be read as prayers. In the poetry sense, these poems are written as examples of patients in recovery.

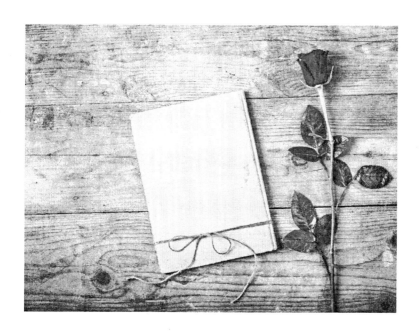

FOUR PRAYERS

A CANCER PATIENT'S PRAYER

Oh dear God,

I haven't talked to you in a while,

but even if I had,

I would still feel like

I had been washed in a turbo washer

and hung out to dry, miles above the earth;

so totally alone,

even though I know you are actually with me,

and I have my family and friends and care team pulling for me.

I hate it when people say

"It's God's will," because I know

that you do not want people

to hurt and get sick;

that's just the way things go in this world.

God, my cancer isn't your fault,

but can you please help me anyway?

I have many, many people and things to live for.

Can you make sure I can stick around for a while?

I want to make a bargain with you,

but that's silly, because what do I have to offer you?

My faith and trust are on a downward slope right now,

they are threatening to disappear

like a rock on a slippery, icy mountain slope.

I also feel like I'm drowning;

please don't let the waters of fear or illness

overtake me.

It's been real hard to pray this, Lord,

because my thoughts wander all over the place;

my head is spinning and my nerves are as tight as strings
on a violin.

I'm ready to explode into a great big puddle.

Please, please take your little girl's hand

and lead her away from the shadow of death.

They say you're walking with me through this valley,

but I don't feel you, God! Please help!

Maybe someday when my thoughts aren't so muddled

you can tell me why this is happening to me.

For now, I imagine me climbing up into your lap

and being rocked to sleep.

I know you care for me, it's just very hard to believe

that right now.

I know you understand. . .

Oh, and one more thing, Lord.

Please keep these people away from me:

the ones who say they know just what I'm going through,

when actually they have never had cancer;

the ones who ask if I need anything but then don't follow through;

also the ones who give me advice about wigs and breast reconstruction

even though they have never had to consider these things.

In trying to be helpful, they say anything they can

think of.

Help me be patient with them; they know not what they do.

Help me to obey my doctor's orders

so that this very long road will not have to be even longer.

Please help your little warrior fight this battle.

Now I lay me down to sleep,

I pray the Lord my soul to keep.

PRAYER IN THREE PERSPECTIVES:

PART ONE

I AM SCARED

Dear God,

Now that I'm dying, I have to make sure I have a good guardian picked out for the kids in case something happens to my husband after I'm gone. Of all things to be worried about as I'm dying, I wish it wasn't necessary to do such careful planning. I was supposed to have a very long life, especially since I was so healthy before the cancer. Well, I guess it goes to show that eating right and exercising don't always keep disease away.

It's been a good life, Lord, but way too short. Now I will never get to see my kids graduate from college or get married or have grandchildren for me to spoil. I hate this dying thing! Why didn't you choose someone else's life to end early? The ones who want to die and are so desperate that they take their own lives. If you let me live, God, I can live in honor of them – really – just trust me, I want to do this – everybody near me wants me to stay with them too. You're so big and powerful, certainly you could work this miracle for me?

I'm scared, Lord, because I'm needing so many naps lately. After I have visitors, I can't even remember who was here. Please let them know I didn't want to be forgetful like this. Everything around me is like a hazy gauze floating around me. Maybe it is angel wings?

I'm scared that I will go into a coma and never come out. I don't know what waits for me on the other side. I hope I can go to heaven, but only you know where I will end up.

Please keep me going until it is time for you to bring to my spiritual home, God. I mean, take me off my painkillers so that I can fully interact with my loved ones at my bedside. Help me to remember the things I need to say to everyone before I pass away.

Will you please take care of my husband and children for me? And when our pets die, could you send them right along to me? I would be so glad to see them.

I put myself into your hands, because I don't know what else to do. Please either make me better or speed up my death, because the not knowing is excruciating. Thank you for listening to my prayer. Amen.

PART TWO

I'M SO SAD

Okay, God, I'm going to tell it to you like it is. Someone once said that you're big and powerful, and you've heard it all before, so you can take anything we say. So, I'm going to talk to you like you're sitting across the table from me.

My friend is dying from cancer, as you know. I am so sad that she is in her final days now, and I am not included in the small group of people that is allowed in the house to see her. I miss her terribly already.

What can I do now? Praying is the only thing I can do, I guess.

She has fought her cancer like a trooper, never giving up, always holding on to her faith. How I wish I had that much faith!

I think when people grieve, we are grieving for ourselves and not the one dying. We are sad we won't see them anymore (unless we see them in heaven later on) and sad to lose a friend. They say death is a part of life, so why does this seem so foreign? I am so utterly helpless, there is nothing left I can do. So powerless! So angry that she has to be taken already!

You know, maybe my friend is the lucky one. She gets to see you and heaven and all her family and friends before I can. She's going where there are no more hurting tears or pain or disabilities or broken hearts. Everything is perfection in heaven, so I'm sure she'll really enjoy it. Thank you, God, for bringing her safely home. Please give me the strength to endure her absence, and help me be thankful she's with you, even though my wishes for the timing of events is not your timing. Help me be a good source of blessing and peace to her family and to do for them what they need right now.

Thank you Lord – Amen.

PART THREE

MY PRAYER FOR THE DYING

Dear God,

I pray for all dying patients,

if they're sad, may the sadness lift;

may they turn to you in their last moments;

may they feel calm in the safety of your hand.

Give the gift of peace from your love

and may they catch a glimpse of you and heaven

ahead of time, to encourage them.

Keep them safe in your care

until it is time for them to finally go home

and see their friends and family

waiting for them on that far shore.

The Lord giveth, and the Lord taketh.

Blessed be the Name of the Lord.

Amen.

FOUR POEMS

IF ONLY

Cancer seems to be on the rise;
so much for living in a modern, educated age

How dare it take us too early
and leave devastation in its wake

If only we could find a cure
cancer would be demolished

We wouldn't have as much to fear
and our losses would be diminished

Let us take a better stand against cancer
do more proactive things for our health

Support patient education against cancer

support the research that is being done

make cancer a thing of the past

I often pray: "Please, oh please, Lord, let it be so."

IN HONOR OF CANCER SURVIVORS

The pronoun "she" used in this poem is a representative word for all cancer survivors.

THE CANCER SURVIVOR WARRIOR

There she is in the grocery store

looking tired and weak.

She is certainly these things,

but her badge of honor is not worn on the outside.

She is much stronger in her character now,

much stronger than she'd ever guess herself to be.

She has been through so much

and probably still forces herself to keep going to her paid job.

There is another cancer survivor in the post office.

You would never guess she has cancer.

She goes about her normal every-day duties

even though she has a membership in "the club."

The cancer survivors club was not something

she ever chose to join,

it just found her as if she won an unseen lottery

that wasn't necessarily genetically based

or inherited.

The lottery "prize" for this club is a sharp wake-up call,

an experience that will teach her things

that she never dreamed she would learn.

The experience changes the warrior's life

forever, but not in a bad way.

Cancer survivors report they receive a new clarity,

a new appreciation for life and their people.

Sometimes membership in the cancer survivors club

leads to a shortened life

and sometimes to a life that has been changed for the better.

Whether her life is cut short or returned to her,

let us remember all the warriors in prayer as they fight for their lives.

Cancer survivors need our support more than

advice we are not qualified to give

and our opinions which mean nothing.

Hats off to my dear fellow members
of the cancer survivors club.
You are awesome and incredibly strong,
brave and courageous.
You may not feel that you are these things,
but someday you will realize it is these qualities
that helped you through.

I pray the Lord would bless you
with good health, guidance and peace.
I am so proud of you,
I love you, and to you I will always
remain loyal and supportive.

ANOTHER DAY

We have an important mission.

There are still breast cancer survivors

Fighting for their lives

and other cancer survivors who passed the hurdle

doing all they can

to raise money for research, education

and patient care.

We have formed an alliance

to let cancer know that we will defeat it.

We know not when, but

it will be done.

All the colored ribbons

Representing other cancers

need our support too.

We need to help others

so they can afford medical care

for their treatment,

and parents won't have to choose
between feeding their kids and getting treatment.
I thank all the corporations for funding research
and helping to raise awareness.

Dear Lord,
I pray for those who are dying from cancer,
that they receive hope and life on earth,
or the ultimate healing in heaven.

Grant them strength and peace
and the same for their families and friends.
We know you're not forgetting us, Lord,
but it's hard to believe sometimes
when things look grim.

We place ourselves in your capable hands
and even if we don't know the outcome,
you do, and you will help us through.
Grant us one more day

and the promise for a better tomorrow.

Amen.

YOU ARE SOMETHING SPECIAL

Abilities we have many,

Talents a few,

and Gifts

one or two.

Abilities help us to survive,

Talents help us to enjoy our lives,

and Gifts help others to enjoy their lives.

Regardless,

we need to realize

there is a plan for each of us.

The abilities, talents, and gifts in our lives

serve a purpose.

In blessing us with them,

God tells us something:

"You are special;

you are loved.

There is no one in the world like you.

I have created you the way I have

for my eternal purposes

and because all your characteristics add up

to be one beloved child of mine.

Do not try to be like someone else,

that would make me sad,

as if you weren't good enough.

But you are exactly what I had in mind for you.

Sure, there are rough edges in you yet,

a cloudy diamond to be polished,

but what work of art doesn't have improvements

made along the way?

In my eyes,

you shine and sparkle

and give me joy.

Please increase my joy further

by not wasting your gifts.

Embrace them and be thankful for them,

for in doing so you honor me.

You are forever in my heart,

and I love you so much,

because you are something special."

EPILOGUE

I hope this little book has helped you. I am thankfully alive after breast cancer, but I am still in the fight to find a cure for all cancers. I will continue to pray against cancer and for the lives of the people who fight against it.

My cancer story is simply one of many who have battled this cancer. I tell you my story to encourage you that you are not alone. Hope can be found, even when things look bleak. I cannot predict how your story will play out, but I do know that somewhere along the way you have a good chance of finding a positive side of cancer.

I want you to know that if I can be of assistance to you or others, I will be glad to keep in touch and help if I can. I love you, dear reader. May God bless you mightily.

INDEX

ABOUT THE AUTHOR

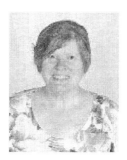

Debbie Loesel Stanton was born in Michigan and has lived in Minnesota for most of her life. She lives in a St. Paul suburb with her husband and with two cats, who are endlessly entertained by the songbirds Debbie feeds outside.

Debbie has always loved the written word, and she furthered that love by creating stories as a child and attempting to write her first book at age 12.

A junior high school teacher submitted a couple of her poems to the local newspaper – although it was publication on a small scale, it encouraged Debbie to continue writing.

After devouring classic poetry in high school, Debbie began to write her own poems. Her love of written verse continues to this day.

Fast forward to 2008: Debbie enrolled in the Christian Writer's Guild two-year online writing course. She completed the first year, then hit a roadblock when she received a breast cancer diagnosis in 2009. Through her experience of surviving cancer came the desire to encourage others not to give up if they got a cancer diagnosis. She subsequently competed the last year of her writing course and later wrote a book about her cancer journey.

The blogging bug caught Debbie in 2012, and she has started several blogs. She has written many stories since then and looks forward to writing even more stories and more books. Living without writing would be an impossibility for her!

E-MAIL: debbielstanton@outlook.com

BLOG: debbiels.com

REVIEWS

The key to a writer's success is the ability to reach readers. There's a lot of work that goes into crafting a message that will resonate with the reading audience, a message that will inform or entertain them.

Readers can also play a big part in helping a book to be discovered. They can review a book so that others can find the book they're looking for. Amazon.com and goodreads.com are good sites that accept book reviews. Reviews can be written by anyone – anonymously if you prefer -- and can include a few words or many.

If you enjoyed my first book, I will be honored if you write a review about it. Thank you in advance for helping me get the word out.

Sincerely,

Debbie Loesel Stanton

BIBLIOGRAPHY